Between Families
and Institutions

Between Families and Institutions

Mental Health and Biopolitical
Paternalism in Contemporary China

ZHIYING MA

Duke University Press   *Durham and London*   2025

© 2025 DUKE UNIVERSITY PRESS. All rights reserved.
Typeset in Warnock Pro by Westchester Publishing Services

Library of Congress Cataloging-in-Publication Data
Names: Ma, Zhiying, [date] author.
Title: Between families and institutions : mental health and
biopolitical paternalism in contemporary China / Zhiying Ma.
Description: Durham : Duke University Press, 2025. | Includes
bibliographical references and index.
Identifiers: LCCN 2024029877 (print)
LCCN 2024029878 (ebook)
ISBN 9781478031741 (paperback)
ISBN 9781478028512 (hardcover)
ISBN 9781478060727 (ebook)
Subjects: LCSH: Mental health policy—China. | Mental health
services—China. | Mental health laws—China. | Community
mental health services—China. | Psychotherapy patients— Family
relationships—China. | Psychiatric hospitals—China.
Classification: LCC RA790.7.C6 M35 2025 (print) | LCC RA790.7.C6
(ebook) | DDC 362.10951—dc23/eng/20250211
LC record available at https://lccn.loc.gov/2024029877
LC ebook record available at https://lccn.loc.gov/2024029878

Cover art: Sophie Hing-Yee Cheung 張馨儀, *Erasing News: Crying
in the Park at Night*, 2023. Newspaper ink and ballpoint pen ink
on erasers, 43.2 × 100 × 1.5 cm. Courtesy of the artist and Ora-Ora
Gallery.

For my parents

Contents

Acknowledgments

This book is owed first and foremost to all my field interlocutors, including people diagnosed with mental illness, their family members, psychiatrists, nurses, social workers, community mental health practitioners, human rights activists, and government officials. They generously shared with me their experiences and perspectives, including their deepest pain and dearest hope. Many welcomed me into their everyday lives, from karaoke parties to clinic visits, and some even used their caregiving or illness experience to help me when my parents and I were ill (which was the subject of a blog I wrote in 2022). To protect their privacy and the privacy of those adjacent to them, I unfortunately cannot name most of my interlocutors, except the following: Dr. Li Jie, Dr. Liang Ju, and Dr. Yao Guizhong were instrumental in helping me gain access to field sites and connecting me to other interlocutors. Ms. Huang Xuetao, Ms. Liu Jiajia, and Dr. Chen Bo invited me to numerous events coordinated by their organization Equity Justice Initiative, where I learned much about the human rights campaign for psychiatric patients' rights. In his eighties and long retired, Dr. Liu Xiehe kindly welcomed me to his home and gave me a precious account of the mental health legislative process. (Note that in this book, when referring to Chinese names, I put the family name first and the given name last, except when the person is a published author in Anglophone academia or media.)

I apologize if my attempts to protect interlocutors' privacy fail to prevent them from receiving unwanted attention or leave anyone feeling unacknowledged. Anonymized or not, I will forever be grateful for the trust, insight, and support of all my interlocutors. Also, any critical analysis offered in this book is aimed not at specific persons but at the discursive and structural conditions that shape their practices. My goals are to change these conditions, help solve the dilemmas facing different stakeholders, and improve mental health services, especially for the benefit of service users and their family members.

Over the years, I have received funding support for the research and writing of this project from various sources. Intramural grants have come from the University of Chicago Division of the Social Sciences, Beijing Center,

Human Rights Program (now the Pozen Center), Urban Network, and William Rainey Harper Fellowship. External grants have come from the Society for Psychological Anthropology/Robert Lemelson Foundation, Association for Asian Studies, Henry Luce Foundation/American Council of Learned Societies, Wuhan University Public Interest and Development Law Institute and Raoul Wallenberg Institute of Human Rights and Humanitarian Law, Ford Foundation, Chiang Ching-kuo Foundation for International Scholarly Exchange, and Wenner-Gren Foundation. Thanks to the Andrew W. Mellon Foundation Research Fellowship, I visited the Needham Research Institute in Cambridge, UK, for three months in 2011 to conduct archival research on the history of madness in China. I am thankful for all the generous funding support and recognition.

My profound gratitude also goes to my graduate mentors at the University of Chicago. Judith Farquhar converted me from psychology to anthropology and tirelessly guided me in my scholarly and personal development over the years. Eugene Raikhel provided me with important orientations in the anthropology of mental health and connected me to many professional development opportunities. Don Kulick's course on vulnerability laid the foundation for my approach to disability and care studies, and his strict mentorship challenged me to become a rigorous scholar. Susan Gal's narrative course gave me the first taste of joy in anthropology; her emphasis on gender and institutional power proved vital not just for this book but also for my new career in social service research. Though not an advisor for my academic research, Richard Taub advocated for my graduate school admission at a time when international students were still rare, and he was always there for a chat when I felt lost. Besides them, I also benefited from the guidance of John Lucy, Julie Chu, Kaushik Sunder Rajan, Johanna Ransmeier, and Jacob Eyferth, among others. Fantastic peers such as Amir Hampel, Michael Chladek, Jason Ingersoll, Jenny Miao Hua, Hiroko Kumaki, Chen Chen, Aaron Seaman, Julia Kowalski, Ender Ricart, and Tal Liron helped me survive graduate school and sharpen my research ideas.

In 2016–2018, I was privileged to be a junior fellow at the Michigan Society of Fellows and an assistant professor at the Department of Anthropology at the University of Michigan–Ann Arbor. The fellowship gave me protected time to start the process of creating this book. I was surrounded with brilliant scholars who pushed me to engage a wider interdisciplinary audience while keeping me grounded in rich ethnographic studies. I especially benefited from conversations with Donald Lopez, Erik Mueggler, Gillian Feeley-Harnik, Andrew Shryock, Krisztina Fehervary, Pedra Kuppers, Mary Gallagher, Liangyu

Fu, Aniket Aga, Kevin Ko, Ana Vinea, Yasmin Moll, Christine Sargent, Ellen Rubenstein, Yun Chen, Jin Li, and Allison Alexy.

After the fellowship, I returned to the University of Chicago to work as a faculty member in the school of social work. My colleagues inspired me to highlight the book's practical implications and social justice commitment. They also formed a crucial social support network for me as I navigated childbirth, parenting, and my father's death. I would especially like to thank Summerson Carr, Robert Chaskin, Colleen Grogan, Yoonsun Choi, Miwa Yasui, Julia Henly, Michele Friedner, Jancey Wickstrom, and Cristina Gros for their mentorship and friendship. Moreover, throughout the years, seasoned administrators such as Anne Ch'ien, Janie Lardner, Linda Turner, Suzanne Fournier, Renee Sibley, Lara Poeppelmeier, and Abbey Newman made the research-related bureaucratic processes smooth sailing. Additionally, Anna Brailovsky's masterful editorship helped me secure important grants.

Beyond these institutions, I relished the feminist and crip (Kim 2017; Rembis 2017) camaraderie of Yige Dong, Mengqi Wang, Yang Zhan, Liat Ben-Moshe, Akemi Nishida, and Alyson Patsavas. Many brilliant scholars gave me invaluable feedback at different stages of the project, including Emily Baum, Amy Borovoy, Paul Brodwin, Howard Chiang, Byron Good, Mary-Jo DelVecchio Good, Susan Greenhalgh, Hsuan-Ying Huang, Jun Jing, Hayden Kantor, Yumi Kim, Andrew Kipnis, Junko Kitanaka, Lisa Richaud, Fabian Simonis, Chao Wang, Li Zhang, and Angela Zito. Benjamin Ross provided thorough copyediting of the manuscript before it was finalized.

I also benefited from engaging conversations with faculty, students, and other audience members in the following meetings and institutions where I was invited to present earlier versions of chapters: the National Academic Conference on Ethical and Legal Issues in Psychiatry, Peking University, China; the Department of Anthropology, Sun Yat-Sen University, China; the "A Better Life Through Science and Biomedicine?" workshop sponsored by the Fairbank Center for Chinese Studies, Harvard University; the Michigan Society of Fellows; the Sociocultural Workshop hosted by the Department of Anthropology, University of Michigan–Ann Arbor; the Madness Afield: Rethinking Psychiatry and Mental Illness in the Non-Western World workshop at the University of California, Irvine; the Disability Studies Program, University of Toledo; the Center for Macau Studies, University of Macau; the Asian American Studies Program, Garrett-Evangelical Theological Seminary; the Forum on the Sociology of Medicine and Health hosted by Southeast University, China; Social Medicine from the South: An Online Mini-Conference, hosted by the Global Social Medicine Network & Wellcome Trust; and the

Scholars Across Anthropology and Social Work workshop; as well as the Clinical Ethnography Workshop, the Medicine, Body, and Practice Workshop, the Institute for the Formation of Knowledge, and the Crown Family School Doctoral Theory Workshop at the University of Chicago.

It was a great pleasure to work with the Duke University Press. I am grateful to my superb editor, Ken Wissoker, for his enthusiasm, sharp vision, and wise guidance for this project, to Ryan Kendall for her outstanding professional assistance in the process, and to the staff at Duke's Editorial, Design, and Production Department and at Westchester Publishing Services for their careful work during the production process. My appreciation also goes to the two anonymous reviewers who read through the manuscript and provided encouraging, incisive, and helpful comments.

A rudimentary overview of this project has been published as "Promises and Perils of *Guan*: Mental Health Care and the Rise of Biopolitical Paternalism in Post-Socialist China," *Medicine Anthropology Theory* 70, no. 2 (September 2020): 150–74. A version of chapter 4 has been published as "Biopolitical Paternalism and Its Maternal Supplements: Kinship Correlates of Community Mental Health Governance in China," *Cultural Anthropology* 35, no. 2 (May 2020): 290–316. A version of chapter 6 has been published as "Affect, Sociality, and the Construction of Paternalistic Citizenship among Family Caregivers in China," *HAU: Journal of Ethnographic Theory* 11, no. 3 (February 2021): 958–71. I thank the editors, reviewers, and copyeditors of those journals for helping to improve my ideas and writing.

Last but certainly not least, I want to thank my family members who accompanied me throughout the entire process, in person or in spirit. My parents developed chronic illnesses while I was in graduate school, but they gave me unflinching support in fieldwork and tolerated me being thousands of miles away when they needed me most. The first-hand experience of my parents and maternal grandparents—I had lost my paternal grandparents by the age of thirteen—with China's drastic transformations and their visceral impact fueled my interest in China Studies and medical anthropology; their innate sense of social justice set the moral compass of my work. Over the past decade, my maternal grandfather, father, and maternal grandmother passed away one after another, but their spirits are with me each day. Finally, my husband, Dongzhou Zhang, gave up his comfortable life in Pasadena and followed me to Chicago early in his graduate studies, only to find me having to leave for fieldwork for a year and a half. After we had our daughter Vida in 2020, he took up many parenting tasks to allow me time to write and work. His love and the joy of having Vida kept me grounded through all the pain, loss, and growth.

Family Ties and Psychiatric Lives

One

One afternoon in fall 2013, I accompanied Mrs. Dong, a woman in her late fifties, to visit her daughter Tingting on a locked psychiatric ward in the southern Chinese city of Nanhua.[1] Two months earlier, Tingting had argued with a colleague and asked her boss for a week's leave to cool off. She had also been turned down by a man she had pursued by buying him many expensive clothes. As Tingting stayed awake night after night and sometimes wandered in the street, Mrs. Dong, who was living with her at the time, grew increasingly worried. With the excuse of a brief check-up to improve her sleep, Mrs. Dong took her to the psychiatric hospital, where she was diagnosed with bipolar disorder and institutionalized.

That fall day, like every other day the previous two months, Mrs. Dong had brought a box of freshly made food, including multigrain porridge, steamed salmon, and stir-fried vegetables, to ensure that her daughter got enough nutrition. Upon seeing us, Tingting, who had been pacing restlessly on the crowded ward, smiled and took the meal box. As soon as she finished eating, however, she demanded that her mother have her released immediately so that she could return to work. "I can't," replied Mrs. Dong, "it's the doctor who makes the decision." This was not true, I thought, for doctors could only *recommend* hospitalization to patients' guardians—in this case, the mother. I kept quiet, suspecting it would be difficult for Tingting to challenge the decision, regardless of who had made it.

Sensing Tingting's irritation, she softened her voice: "Don't worry. I've planned out everything after your discharge." It turned out that she had sent a resignation letter to Tingting's company and had bought a small storefront near their home so that they could run an herbal tea stall together. As Mrs. Dong saw it, Tingting's workplace was too stressful of an environment. In fact, any job that required Tingting to work "outside" on her own would probably expose her to undue stress, unhealthy food, or troublesome relationships. The tight work schedule would also prevent her from adhering to her medications. "Well, from now on life will be more relaxing for you," Mrs. Dong announced with a beam.

"NO!" Tingting screamed, "I'm 30 years old. I'm not a kid anymore. Why do you want to control (管/*guan*) me when I'm supposed to be independent? Before I was sent here, I had been sorting out the clothes, my work, and my moods. I only needed some more time. You threw me in here and that totally messed me up. Please, leave me alone!"

"You're sick, Tingting," sighed Mrs. Dong. "How can I leave you alone (不管你/*buguan ni*)?"

Two

On May 6, 2013, forty-seven-year-old Xu Wei filed suit against his eldest brother and a psychiatric hospital in Shanghai where he had stayed for thirteen years, asking to be released.[2] He claimed that in his twenties, he had traveled to Australia to learn English and work. To earn his tuition, he tried his luck at a casino, where he became addicted to drugs. Failing to renew his visa, he had to return to Shanghai and live with his father. He overcame his drug addiction but soon started feeling that he was being followed. His father took him to the district mental health center, where he was diagnosed with schizophrenia and kept for a year. After his release, he fought with his father over work-related issues and accidentally injured him.[3] His father had him committed again, this time at a run-down hospital on the outskirts of the city (Xishu 2018).

In the hospital, Wei initially attempted suicide by jumping out of a fifth-floor window, but that only fractured his bones. Then he fell in love with a female patient, and they repeatedly tried to escape in the hope of building a family together. Once, they ran as far as the city's train station, only to be intercepted by the hospital staff. After that incident, the woman's family agreed to have her released if Wei was as well. Some doctors at the hospital also thought that Wei was stable enough to live outside, so they reached out to Xu Xing, Wei's eldest brother and guardian since their father's death, to see if he would be willing to sign the release papers. Xing worked in another province and seldom visited Wei. In fact, even Wei's hospitalization was paid for with his own public medical insurance and welfare benefits. Nevertheless, Xing rejected Wei's release, saying, "I'm his guardian! I have to watch over (*guan*) him. I have to be responsible for society!"

Wei suspected that Xing had an ulterior motive: they had inherited their father's two apartments together and Xing had been collecting rent, so he probably did not want to share the profits. The hospital staff turned to Wei's neighborhood committee and other relatives to see if any were willing to become his guardian instead and authorize his release. They all said no, except for Wei's mother, who had divorced Wei's father and left the family three decades before. In early 2012, she filed a request to the district court, hoping to replace Xing as Wei's guardian. The court rejected her request, citing her old age as a concern (Chen 2016b).

Wei did not give up. Browsing the internet with his smartphone, he found Huang Xuetao, a Shenzhen-based and nationally renowned human rights advocate for psychiatric patients. I first learned of Wei's struggles in an online discussion about the district court's ruling that Huang had organized. In the discussion, a law student questioned: "The district court said that Wei's brother had fulfilled his responsibility as a guardian. Does this mean that parents can just lock their children up in psychiatric hospitals, rent out their homes, and go to work elsewhere?"

"Well, the court simply wanted to make sure that the patient was 'carefully watched over' (小心看管/*xiaoxin kanguan*). Those are the exact words in every local mental health regulation throughout the country," another law student explained.

A bewildered social worker then asked: "But patients are humans, not objects, right?"

Shortly after that discussion, Huang found Wei a local attorney to file a lawsuit for him. The filing took place mere days after the first national Mental Health Law (MHL) in China had come into effect on May 1, 2013. The law was groundbreaking in that it declared that people with mental illness are sovereign individuals with rights to autonomy in both hospitalization and discharge. As the case progressed, I visited Wei in his hospital. When we talked, scores of inmates looked at us from afar, and a few approached us to listen in, eyes glistening with hope and curiosity. I asked Wei how he felt about the prospects of his case. He briefly smiled and then blankly stared ahead:

"You know, my brother neglects (不管/*buguan*) me, and I'm like a ball being kicked around . . . When it comes down to it, there has to be someone willing to take responsibility."

At the Crossroads of Madness, Family, and Institutions

For the past few decades in China, people diagnosed with serious mental illnesses (SMIs) have been automatically placed under the guardianship of their close relatives, including spouses, parents, adult children, and siblings. According to a practice called "medical protection hospitalization" that was prevalent until the MHL, a psychiatrist might advise that a patient be hospitalized, and then the guardian would "decide whether to accept the advice or not, and when to finish or withdraw from the hospitalization and treatment" (Shao et al. 2010, 5). A survey has indicated that as of 2003, about 60 percent of psychiatric inpatients in China were admitted by their family members against their will (Pan, Xie, and Zheng 2003). Another survey conducted in a major psychiatric hospital in Southern China shows that 64.6 percent of people who had been hospitalized there for over a year could not be discharged because of their family members' refusals (Luo et al. 2014). Meanwhile, patients' medical treatment, involuntary or otherwise, is typically paid for by their families or by public medical insurance and other welfare subsidies their families have scrambled together. Outside of the hospital, over 90 percent of people diagnosed with SMIs live with, and are supported by, their families (Phillips 1993).

In this context, the two opening stories, which I will continue to unpack in subsequent chapters, are far from unique. Instead, they reveal how Chinese families are entangled in mental health care and its institutional processes. On one end, Tingting's story represents the beginning of such entanglements, where people view their loved ones' everyday life problems—love, work, money, and so on—as mental illness and seek help from psychiatry. On the other end, Xu Wei's story points to a plateau of such entanglements, where the guardian may view the patient as the problem who requires constant management through indefinite hospitalization. One may ask: How do these translations happen? How do they shape the contours of kin responsibility, compelling people to alter the futures of their loved ones as well as their own? On what grounds do people claim or contest the authority to do so? How might patient management blur the lines between care, control, and abandonment? How does it make or break family ties and people's senses of sociopolitical belonging?

Families' entanglements in psychiatry have been brought into sharp relief by relevant policies and regulations, especially the recent mental health legal reform. Starting in 2006, human rights activists such as Huang Xuetao campaigned forcefully against widespread involuntary hospitalization in China, families' involvement in it, and the country's oppressive culture of paternalism supposedly undergirding these phenomena. In response, psychiatrists who had drafted the MHL defended these practices as manifestations of "state paternalism" (国家父权/guojia fuquan), which presumably provided "care and love for the sick, the vulnerable, and the disabled even against their own will" (Xie and Ma 2011b). These debates expedited the passage of the MHL, which had been in the making for nearly three decades. As mentioned, the 2013 MHL affirms patient autonomy and the voluntary principle of hospitalization. Curiously, it also upholds families' guardianship of patients. In particular, it grants guardians the rights to consent to patients' treatment and to hospitalize against their will any patients who pose actual or potential danger to themselves or others. Meanwhile, it stipulates that families have the responsibility to provide for, look after, and monitor patients (National People's Congress 2012). Thus, the family, as it has been conceived in the MHL, has become a primary unit to mediate the individual liberty, well-being, and population security of the nation. One may ask: How was the idea of family guardianship justified in the legislation process? How does it interact with notions of freedom, authority, rights, and responsibility in discourse and practice? How does the law shape the fate of people like Xu Wei and the country's landscape of mental health care?

All these questions boil down to a simple inquiry: *why has the family occupied such a critical role in Chinese psychiatry, especially during the recent mental health legal reform?* This is the central question of my book. Some readers might see this as a non-question, arguing that the Confucian culture has long determined Chinese families' entrenchment in the care of members with mental illness (Lin and Lin 1980). Nevertheless, historical examinations that I present later in this chapter show constant change in such involvement and its conceptualization.

In this book, I analyze families' involvement in medicine as shifting technological, institutional, and ideological configurations. Note that *configure* here means both to represent by an image and to fashion or compile in a certain form, because how these forces represent the family also shapes how they interact with, intervene into, and regulate it. These configurations are co-constituted with how people in and beyond the household think of madness and normality, how they define and distribute responses to vulnerability and disruptions, their desired order of life and society, and the perceived expertise and power of medicine in achieving that order. Therefore, by tracing an entangled and emergent history of madness, family, medicine, and related laws and policies in China, this book provides a fuller understanding of the affects, ethics, and political economy of care and population governance in China.

Drawing on extended fieldwork as well as archival and media analysis, this book shows that in contemporary China, psychiatric knowledge, together with the state's growing security concerns, constructs people diagnosed with SMIs as chronically risky subjects requiring perpetual, intimate management. In the mental health legal reform and other policy discussions, policymakers have used China's historical legacies and cultural ethics of paternalism to frame measures of patient management as care that the state undertakes for its people. Meanwhile, as paternalistic values circulate from the state to medical professionals and then to families, actual responsibilities for care and management end up falling to families, particularly women and the elderly. This ideological legitimation and structural displacement of biomedically defined responsibilities of population management constitute what I refer to as *biopolitical paternalism*. It produces a wide variety of conflicts and harm within families and aggravates health disparities across the mentally ill population. Yet tensions between the ideological legitimation and structural displacement of biopolitical paternalism also allow people to flip the script (Carr 2010), calling on the state to be a proper parent for its vulnerable children.

Though discovered in mental health, biopolitical paternalism bespeaks the general tenor of governance in contemporary China, given the widespread reconfiguration of the revolutionary "people" into a biologized "population" to be managed (Cho 2010; Dutton 2005), the neoliberal devolution of welfare and health care, and the rise of the security state (Lee and Zhang 2013). Throughout the world in years past, many states promised or enacted paternalistic care for their citizens (Shever 2013; Verdery 1996); now they have similarly relegated responsibilities of care to families and other intimate/

informal relationships (Biehl 2005; Eichner 2017), while expecting or de-manding them to act as private paternalistic agents to manage individuals deemed vulnerable or deviant (Soss, Fording, and Schram 2011). Beyond the nation states, international humanitarian and human rights organizations also often impose what they think is good on marginalized communities through a mix of care and control (Barnett 2017). Thus, the concept of biopo-litical paternalism helps us detect, in different governance mechanisms, how subjects are constituted and regulated; how responsibilities for care and management are legitimized, distributed, and implemented; and the power effects of these mechanisms.

Historicizing and Politicizing the Family

The Advent of Psychiatry and the Essentialization of Chinese Families

While a historical approach will run through this book, a glance at how fam-ilies were configured in relation to madness/mental illness before and after the advent of psychiatry in China will start destabilizing the seeming natu-ralness and inevitability of current practices. For most of the imperial era, a common phenomenology of madness was 乱/*luan*, or chaotic words and behavior. Rather than being located solely in the mind, it was thought to re-flect entangled physiological, emotional, and social processes that disrupted the normal flow of life force (气/*qi*). Thus, physicians of Chinese medicine prescribed drugs to restore a patient's organic balance or pacify disordered emotions (Zhang 2007). They might also help establish proper social roles and relations for the person, such as instructing relatives to find a spouse for someone who was thought to be maddened by unfulfilled sexual desires (Simonis 2010). At any rate, because the behavioral, emotional, and social chaos was apparent, and because the physiological disruptions could be di-agnosed with medical skills, physicians did not have to rely on the person's relatives to uncover any hidden illness. Because madness was typically seen as a temporary aberrance, families were not expected to make any long-term special arrangements for the person, either at home or somewhere else.

There were also no specific legal arrangements for mad persons in most of the imperial era. Matters began to change when a 1667 Qing law exonerated mad persons who had committed homicide because of their lack of intention, while it required their relatives to compensate the victims' families. As officials came to see madness as a disorder with potential homicidal impulses, they began to fear the dangerousness of all mad persons. A 1732 rule required families to declare any insane member to the local government. In 1766, another rule required relatives to manage (*guan*) the mad persons and restrain them in a safe room, and local officials were to issue locks and chains so that confinement could be strictly implemented. If home confinement was not well enforced and the mad person committed homicide, the relatives would be harshly sentenced (Simonis 2010).

While the medical and popular discourses saw madness as a temporary, curable disorder, the law now saw madness as a permanent threat to society. By requiring the family to control and confine the person, the law sought to turn the family into a disciplinary agent. At any rate, recorded cases of (long-term) confinement were few, both before and after the Qing legal stipulation. As historian Fabien Simonis (2010) suggested, "what the government came to see as the most dangerous aspect of madness (its unpredictable intermittency) was precisely what many people considered the best reason not to declare a mad relative" (465). Many families ignored the legal stipulation and unchained the periodically mad persons because they saw them as having recovered from temporary madness or because they needed the labor for agricultural work.

In 1898, John G. Kerr, an American Presbyterian missionary doctor, opened the first refuge for the insane in China in the city of Canton (now Guangzhou). He did so mostly with his own financial resources, because other medical missionaries either had deemed the insane persons incorrigible or seen the seemingly serene oriental culture as more suitable to care for them than the high-strung Western civilization. To justify the establishment of the refuge, Kerr and his colleagues often discussed the confinement and other abuses that Chinese families inflicted on insane persons. For example, he stated: "Among the better classes, confinement in a strong room, and often loaded with chains, was all that could be done. A short method of getting rid of the hopelessly incurable has no doubt often been adopted in a country where the father holds the power of life and death over his family, and death has been hastened among the poorer classes by the want of care and ill-treatment" (Kerr 1898, 177). Kerr was generalizing from the cases he had observed, and he was probably projecting on China the Roman legal tradition that had allowed *pater familias* or household heads absolute power over other members (Harders 2012). It was a projection because the Confucian concept of filiality actually assumed reciprocal rather than unilateral responsibilities in hierarchical relations by emphasizing the gratitude that one should have toward one's parents for their nurturance (Zito 1997). At any rate, depictions like this framed Chinese families as spaces of harm reflecting the oppressive Chinese culture; they also framed the refuge as a safe space that could rescue and enlighten the insane person as an individual rather than as part of the filial relations. Before long, the discourse of liberating the insane from home confinement had gained dominance among medical missionaries, and they established similar asylums in several other Chinese cities.

By presenting home confinement as a problem inherent to the Chinese family, medical missionaries ignored how the Qing government had mandated it as well as how families had negotiated with or even resisted this mandate. Such omissions in turn allowed them to accept requirements to confine the insane from the local government without critical self-reflection. By 1904, the Kerr Refuge (as it came to be known) had started to admit patients sent and paid for by the police department, and the staff saw this as a sign of official recognition (Selden 1910). By 1909, half of its patients were supported by the government, many of whom had been picked up from the street (Selden 1909a). Along this process, staff at the Refuge built thicker walls to prevent patients from escaping (Selden 1909b) and devised tools such as wire restraining frames to contain them (Ross 1920). Through its government collaboration, missionary psychiatry became a control mechanism, and it began to treat the insane person as a subject of discipline rather than as a universal human.

Inspired by the Kerr Refuge and asylums abroad, the Qing government established an asylum in Beijing in 1908, where social deviants such as vagabonds who had been deemed insane were not so much treated as they were policed and provided for (Baum 2018). Then in the 1910s and 1920s, influenced by Euro-American eugenic thought, some medical missionaries came to see the insane person as a biological body carrying hereditary defects and moral degeneracy, threatening the health of the population (Hofmann 1913).[4] Interestingly, while missionaries criticized Chinese family customs for worsening the heredity of future generations by expecting everyone to marry and reproduce, they also sought to harness the reproductive drive of the Chinese family for eugenic purposes. For instance, they urged the family to heed "stock and seed selection" by investigating the reproductive history of a concubine before taking her in (Ross 1926, 10). As such, missionary psychiatry began to treat the Chinese family as both an object and an ally of intervention, useful for the purposes of population improvement.

Guided by the eugenics discourse, the Republican national and local governments issued laws that mandated the institutionalization of all insane persons and that forbade people from having sex with them (Woods 1923).

Families distressed by war and poverty learned to send their members to the asylum for medical attention and temporary relief (Baum 2018). All these developments were halted and the field severely disrupted by the Sino-Japanese War and the subsequent Chinese Civil War. Around 1949, when the People's Republic was founded, there were only six hundred psychiatric beds and fewer than fifty psychiatrists across the country. Most of these resources were concentrated in five (some report nine) major municipal psychiatric hospitals (Pearson 1995, 11), all in a state of disrepair using only barebones treatment and constraint. Yet the ways psychiatry essentialized and problematized Chinese families' role in causing, treating, and managing madness, along with the ways such configurations enabled the field's development and collaboration with state power, left a lasting legacy that is still impactful today.

The Family and the State, in and beyond Chinese History

Configurations of the family are important not just for the development of psychiatry but also for arrangements of politics and economics (Franklin and McKinnon 2001). In imperial China, filiality was an "organizing trope for connecting cosmic and social hierarchies" in Confucianism (Zito 1997, 58); that is, the father-son relationship was supposed to be a model for relationships between the heavens and humans, lord and subject, and so on. Since the imperial order collapsed at the turn of the twentieth century, nation building and state governance projects have repeatedly mobilized ideas of, and practices from, the family to reconstruct meanings of personhood, state-society relations, and the relationship between tradition and modernity (Barlow 1993). For instance, similar to the contemporaneous medical missionaries, leaders of the 1910s "New Culture Movement" traced many evils of traditional Chinese society to the Confucian patriarchy, contending that it had subjected individuals to inhumane moral codes and outright oppression. From then on, public discourses were suffused with the metaphor of breaking the "iron cage of the feudal family" to achieve individual freedom (Lee 2007). The Nationalist (1912–1949) and Maoist (1949–late 1970s) governments both launched campaigns and policies to fight manifestations of patriarchal oppression such as polygamy and arranged marriages (Glosser 2003). However, because these campaigns sought to strengthen the nation-state, they again emphasized the importance of the family for individual and social development (Stacey 1983). Of course, the Maoist regime did, to an extent, downplay the role of households and instead organized citizens into collectives, including urban work units and rural communes.

In the market reform era following Mao's death, government and public discourses have come to blame collectivization for having produced socioeconomic apathy. They celebrate the family as an essential social unit that simultaneously propels the market economy and provides individuals with a haven because of people's putatively natural desire for a good life for themselves and their loved ones. This turn to the family—or what Yunxiang Yan (2018) has called "neo-familism"—has been accompanied and conditioned by the state's withdrawal from the provision of social welfare. For example, the 1996 Law on the Protection of the Rights and Interests of the Elderly stipulated that "the elderly shall be provided for mainly by their families" (National People's Congress 1996, Article 10), just as state-owned enterprises in urban areas laid off workers en masse and canceled their retirement pensions. Note that the state has not simply retreated from the family; rather, its institutional powers have seeped into family life to produce what it sees as normal, desirable subjects. The most famous example is the one-child policy (1982–2015), which made the married couple a key site of population control and allowed the state to directly intervene into women's reproductive choices (Greenhalgh 2008).

As ideas of the family have been used to shore up various forms of political order, the ensuing social transformations have in turn reshaped the structure and power dynamics of families. Existing research has shown that in late imperial China, the ideal-typical family structure was a patriarchy, characterized by "patrilineal descent and inheritance, patrilocal residence, strong parental authority, and the power of the senior generation (particularly but not exclusively senior males) reinforced by state law and property ownership" (Harrell and Santos 2017, 8). Over the twentieth century, forces like war and urbanization continued to reduce family size and paternal authority. Especially after the establishment of the People's Republic, economic reconstructions, mass education, and the revolutionary ideology boosted women's labor participation rate, raising their status both within and outside of the home. Since the 1980s, ideas of privacy and privatization have increased the appeal of conjugal intimacy and nuclear families (Yan 1997), while the one-child policy has made childrearing the focus of the household (Fong 2004; Kuan 2015; Xu 2017). In recent years, the state's renewed endorsement of Confucian values has exacerbated male domination at home and beyond, while the growing burden of family care has in turn driven many women out of the workforce to become full-time caregivers (Evans 2017).

The extant scholarship has shown how families exist as ideological and institutional constructs, fields of intimate politics, or units of survival and care in times of rapid social transformation. This book brings these dimensions together and illuminates their interconnections by exploring the dynamics between family life and professional expertise, institutions, and law (Kowalski 2016; Povinelli 2006) and by focusing on situations of severe illness and vulnerability, when people's deepest senses of dignity, responsibility, and attachment are at stake (Mattingly 2014). For example, chapter 1 continues to trace how medical discourses, social policies, and the broader political economy have aligned to configure the role of the family in mental health care in the People's Republic, culminating in a hospital-family circuit where patients are bound and kin guardianship is enshrined. Chapter 3 examines how risks and responsibilities highlighted by the psychiatric discourse of SMI intersect with market forces to rework family relations, rendering some ties impossible and others more fragile. Note that sometimes people turn to ties not recognized by the guardianship system—such as an aunt or an unmarried partner—for intimacy and care. This book will examine these "found" or "chosen" families, exploring how they are assembled and what the lack of legal and policy recognition means to them.

Front and center in my multidimensional analysis of the family is gender. After all, as anthropologists of kinship have reminded us, gender helps articulate systems of meaning and mediates pathways of inequality in and beyond the household (Yanagisako and Collier 1987). For instance, although the guardianship system grants family members paternalistic authority in patient management, the fact that aging women are often the primary caregivers means that their exercise of such authority is at best precarious; we can see this in Mrs. Dong's eagerness to deny any power she had in deciding whether or not Tingting would be discharged. Meanwhile, compared to other family members and professionals, these women's vulnerability and proximity to patients may make them more compassionate and more willing to accommodate desires and habits that seem strange or are not approved by psychiatry (chapters 3 and 4). Thus, another dimension of the family less discussed in the literature is a source of improvisation on, and resistance to, officially endorsed subjectivities and relations.

As the title suggests, this book interrogates the complex relationships and productive tensions between familial intimacy and institutional powers. With the term *institutions*, some readers may think of what sociologist Erving Goffman (1961) called "total institutions"—that is, enclosed spaces where groups of people lead formally registered lives, such as closed-door psychiatric hospitals. While these hospitals certainly dominate the landscape of mental health care in China, institutions also include other formal organizations designed, tasked, and contracted by the government to regulate aspects of society, such as community mental health teams and social work agencies in our case. In this sense, family lives are shaped by an array of institutions whose work may or may not be aligned with each other, and this can reveal the effects of their power. Moreover, if we expand the definition of institutions to include recurring practices that enforce norms, facilitate/constrain behavior, and give people identities (Martin 2004), then families are institutions vital for producing and managing individual subjects. Because the family can be seen either as a basic social institution or as a pristine private realm, it affords various imaginations of the state and enables people to constantly draw, redraw, and contest the state's boundaries. Finally, as family members face vulnerability and precarity together, they may deviate from the teachings of governing institutions and engage with each other, as well as the broader society and state, in non-normative ways. These disruptions and improvisations may in turn bring changes to the state and its institutions. Across the world, the family is typically regarded as the most ordinary aspect of people's lives. Meanwhile, "family values"—whatever they are—are used to facilitate and define various forms of body politic (McKinnon and Cannell 2013). Therefore, these dynamics and tensions are relevant far beyond mental health and China.

Madness, Biopolitics, and Care

Constructing and Experiencing Madness/Mental Illness

Like the family, madness/mental illness is a shifting social construct.[5] Since the nineteenth century, psychiatry in Euro-American countries has come to see atypical human feelings and behavior from a disease-specific lens (Rosenberg 2007). Then, since the 1950s, psychiatry has been increasingly dominated by biomedicalization—that is, the reduction of mental illnesses to neurochemical disorders that require treatment with psychopharmaceuticals. In this process, talk therapies and other healing approaches have been separated out and largely deemed inferior (Luhrmann 2011). Many Western scholars have criticized biomedical psychiatry as a form of social control: the behavioral norms that it shores up deny human diversity, the biological reductionism helps to conceal the social injustice that produces distress in the first place (Laing 1965), and the medical treatment falsely claims competence in addressing people's everyday problems (Szasz 1964). Moreover, they argue that the coercive measures deployed by psychiatry—particularly involuntary hospitalization and forced medication—strip people of autonomy, moral responsibility, and opportunities for personal growth, subjecting them to stigma, oppression, and social death (Cooper 1971; Goffman 1961).[6]

In China, more than a century since medical missionaries built the first asylum for the insane, biomedical psychiatry has become an established field. Despite China's recent *psycho-boom*—the growing popularity of the use of counseling and psychological self-help among the public (Huang 2015; Zhang 2020), those resources are not typically available or seen as appropriate for persons diagnosed with SMIs. Instead, medication and hospitalization have become two dominant modes of service for them. This book addresses how meanings of disorder, chronicity, and risk are constructed on the closed psychiatric ward (chapter 2), at home (chapter 3), and in emerging community mental health practices (chapter 4).[7] Inspired by existing critiques of psychiatry, I face the hegemony of biomedicalized and institutionalized psychiatry in China head on, asking what social will it helps to establish (Lovell and Rhodes 2014) and what impact it has on people with lived experience.

While most critiques of psychiatry that have emerged from Western liberal societies concern social constructions of madness and the individual's experience with oppression,[8] I emphasize the dynamic and diverse ways in which madness/mental illness is relationally constructed and experienced—how people identify and understand madness in household life, how they come to desire psychiatric treatment for their loved ones, how psychiatry defines itself by imagining and intervening into family care, and how people draw on, reframe, resist, or supplement psychiatric ideas in everyday familial interactions. Along the way, I will compare the practices in China with those that scholars have noticed in other Asian and Latin American countries, where families are also enmeshed in psychiatry (e.g., Nakamura 2013; Pinto 2014; Reyes-Foster 2018; Rubinstein 2018). At first glance, one major difference seems to be Chinese families' routine use of hospitalization and the legal expectation of it.

As mentioned, this book focuses on people diagnosed with SMIs. In China, the term *serious mental illnesses* is an administrative category, covering schizophrenia, bipolar disorder, paranoid disorder, schizoaffective disorder, epilepsy with psychosis, and intellectual disability with psychosis (Ministry of Health 2012), with the first two diagnoses being the most common in my fieldwork. These individuals are typically called "patients" by service providers, family members, government officials, the public, and even themselves. I struggled with whether to use this term in my writing, because it might risk reinforcing medicalization and equating persons with pathologies.

Nevertheless, alternatives preferred by people who encounter psychiatry in Euro-American contexts—most notably *consumers, survivors,* and *service users*—are much less used or even understood in China outside a small circle of advocates. Further, these terms carry their own assumptions—such as the individual's power to choose and the history of open confrontations with institutions—that may not be applicable in our case (Speed 2006). Therefore, I have decided to keep the term *patients,* not to endorse any biomedical reductionism but to track how discourses and practices around it shape personal experiences, such as the restricted choices these individuals face. In fact, because many people refuse to see themselves as having mental illness (chapter 1), using the term *patient* can illustrate how the label is imposed and contested. To reflect these contestations around the truth status of mental illness and to keep the possibilities open, I will also refer to "people *diagnosed* with SMIS" instead of "people with SMIS" whenever appropriate.

Meanwhile, taking a constructivist approach to mental illness does not mean denying individuals' suffering and vulnerability. The suffering and vulnerability are real, whether as a result of bodily processes, traumatizing relationships, social injustice, or the looping effects of psychiatric labeling and institutional segregation (Hacking 2000). This book attends to individuals' help-seeking attempts sympathetically, while analyzing how they are molded by the existing mental health-care system. For instance, the limited venues and modalities of mental health services, coupled with the privatization of health care, mean that families who cannot afford these services are often without help and that psychiatry—however problematic—may be highly appealing to them and sometimes to patients themselves. As scholars and activists seeking to promote the well-being of patients and their loved ones, we need to simultaneously confront psychiatric coercion while acknowledging the lived reality of vulnerability to understand how psychiatric hegemony and health-care shortages coexist and are mediated by intimate relations.

Between Biopower and Care

Through their involvement in mental health services, family members typically see themselves as taking on responsibilities for vulnerable others (Levinas 1988) and exploring visions of the good life (Mol, Moser, and Pols 2010). As such, their actions could be understood through the lens of care. Feminist scholars have long argued that, unlike the assumption of free, equal, and independent individuals dominant in Western liberal thinking, human beings are inherently vulnerable and dependent—though to varying degrees;

as such, care is and should be recognized as the basis of social life (Kittay 1999; Ruddick 1995; Tronto 1993). Empirically, anthropologists have examined which lived moral experiences drive people to care (Kleinman 2009a; Mattingly 2014) and what prevents care (Scheper-Hughes 1993). They have also examined how care is shaped by different ethical frameworks (Stonington 2020) and how it is achieved through routinized actions (Aulino 2016). Inspired by these works, this book interrogates how care is conceptualized in professional knowledge, law, and social policies; how it is shaped by different socioeconomic conditions and service access; and how people attend to their loved ones' needs and desires through words, actions, and material arrangements amid all these forces. Because the personhood of those diagnosed with SMIs is often in question, I also address what kind of moral agency (Myers 2015) family care might afford them and how it might affect their recovery and social inclusion.

While the public tends to assume that care is transparent, apolitical, and naturally loving,[9] the opening vignettes have shown that family actions are more complex than that. After all, the psychiatric services in which families are involved—and implicated—are a mechanism of biopower, for they turn the supposedly "basic biological features of the human species," in particular the risks that mental illnesses pose to patients and the public, into "the object of a political strategy, of a general strategy of power" (Foucault 2009, 1). While most studies of biopower have focused on how formal institutions, professional experts, or the knowledge they instill serve to discipline the individual body or regulate the population, some anthropologists have examined how families in different societies are entangled in the exercise of biopower (e.g., Biehl 2005; Friedman 2008; Stevenson 2014). Bearing this in mind, this book explores how biopower is performed by nonexperts in intimate relations and how the family may work as a model, a site, an instrument, or a product of biopower in contemporary China.[10]

Connecting these two concepts, this book illustrates how biopower requires, enables, inhibits, and transforms different forms of care. On the one hand, in the mental health legislation process, leading psychiatrists and policymakers did envision involuntary hospitalization as benevolent care, precisely because it could supposedly temper patients' risks of illness relapse and violent behavior (chapter 1). A preoccupation with public security risk also prompted the state's investment in developing countrywide community mental health services (chapter 4). In everyday life, psychiatry's promises of normality and order give family members hope, and as we saw in Tingting's case, one of the ways the mother expressed concern for the daughter was to ensure her medication compliance. Thus, care and biopower may be mutually constituted: while biopower sets the goal of care and utilizes people's intimate practices to realize itself, care may be achieved through techniques of biopower.[11]

On the other hand, as biopower transforms family members' desire to care into a mandate of risk management, it may produce or exacerbate conflicts between people receiving and giving such care, inflicting harm on both sides. To secure professional services for their loved ones, family members may find it necessary to adopt and manipulate the category of risk; as they become more attuned to risk, some family members—such as Xu Wei's brother—may choose to have patients hospitalized indefinitely, thereby depriving their social membership (chapter 5). Of course, family members may engage in many other practices to nurture patients' holistic being and to repair the damages wreaked by medication and hospitalization, but such practices are typically dismissed or denounced by psychiatrists.

An analysis of these diverse familial actions and decisions can reveal how epistemological and ethical boundaries between good and bad care—or between care, control, and abandonment—can be fragile and contentious (Pinto 2014) and how such contentions are "coproduced by high-order mandates as well as the local context of practice" in biopower (Brodwin 2012, 15). In this book, when I use the word *caregivers* to refer to family members who assume responsibilities to make arrangements for patients, I fully acknowledge and seek to highlight these contentions.

Guan and the Ethics/Politics of Paternalism

Our two opening stories show how ethical contentions are often registered in the Chinese word 管/*guan*. In Chinese, a single character often constitutes a word in and of itself. Many single-character words are polysemic; that is, they have two or more somewhat related meanings, and only the context in which they are uttered can specify their meaning-in-use. Single characters can also be combined to construct less ambiguous compound words. Depending on the context and the word combination, *guan* can refer to concern for and responsibility toward another individual or to managing, governing, intervening, and control. For example, in the first story, the same actions—the mother hospitalizing the daughter against her will, planning her future, protecting her from potential harm, and ensuring her medical compliance—was seen as control by the daughter but as care by the mother, and both interpretations were expressed in *guan*. As such, *guan* constitutes a keyword whose polysemy "both reflect[s] and influence[s] the processes of contention over ideas and values" (Kipnis 2006, 295; see also Williams 1985).

Despite its polysemy, *guan* has an entrenched meaning for many Chinese speakers—that is, the ethical practice of parenting. As cultural psychologists and anthropologists have told us, when Chinese parents practice *guan* with their children, their seemingly stern behavior of control, discipline, and restraint is often accompanied by care, love, and sacrificial labor (Xu 2017). Underlying these practices is an image of children as "weak, vulnerable, and dependent beings" (Saari 1990, 8) who have to be protected and trained in an optimal environment by their more mature and knowledgeable parents. Parents engage in *guan* with the hope that their children can become fully human (成人/*chengren*), act in harmony with the social order (Chao 1994), and eventually no longer need *guan*. Because this *guan* seamlessly connects individual development, parental aspirations, and social order, scholars have argued that *guan* is "the characteristic feature of Chinese socialization" (Wu 1996, 14). Seen in this light, the contention between Tingting and her mother was partly about whether it would be appropriate to apply *guan* to an adult who should have become a full human enjoying relative autonomy or whether madness had turned the adult into a vulnerable, child-like being requiring *guan*.

As we saw in Tingting's story, contentions around *guan* also pertain to how it is practiced with psychiatric techniques and institutional arrangements. This book shows that psychiatrists, community mental health practitioners, and local officials often invoke the language of *guan* as they teach family members to monitor patients' symptoms, risks, and pharmaceutical compliance. Moreover, *guan* has dominated the legal and policy texts produced and promoted by the Central government. In particular, the new MHL highlights *guan* as a principle of mental health work, with the term taking on a specific meaning as management (管理/*guanli*). Interestingly, while the law opens by requiring "all facets of society" to participate in *guan* or comprehensive management of people diagnosed with SMIs (National People's Congress 2012, Article 6), it quickly relegates most of this responsibility to their families. Article 21 of the law stipulates: "If it appears that a family member may have a mental disorder, other family members shall help them obtain prompt medical care, provide for their daily needs, and assume responsibility for their supervision and management (*guanli*)."

This book traces the circulation of *guan* between family practices, psychiatric encounters, policy discussions, and legal reform.[12] Acknowledging its polysemy, I explore how people define, evaluate, and contest *guan* in different realms; how family members' desire to parent, to care for the vulnerable, and to search for order are transformed when *guan* is mobilized, emphasized, and reconfigured by medical and legal discourses; and the power effects of these processes on various actors and relations. For instance, when *guan* is reconfigured as a mandate for families to perpetually manage patients' risks using any means, including indefinite hospitalization, it not only exerts heavy constraints on people like Xu Wei but also contradicts their understanding of *guan*, which is hinged on intimate relations, kindred affects, and the production of hope (chapter 5).

While people from all walks of life use the keyword *guan* to express ideas about how mental illness should be dealt with and how families should be involved, psychiatrists, policymakers, and human rights activists also use the keyword *paternalism* to articulate the logics behind their positions. After all, *guan* is commonly seen as an exercise of parental—and especially paternal—authority, responsibility, and wisdom. During the mental health legislative debates, both human rights activists and psychiatrists who drafted the law framed involuntary hospitalization as a manifestation of paternalism, which both sides viewed as a defining feature of the Chinese family, state, and culture; their contention was in whether this paternalism was oppressing or protecting people and whether it should be overthrown or endorsed. In this book, I acknowledge the actors' views while critically analyzing the historical formations, contemporary meanings, and practical operations of paternalism as it undergirds mental health care and governance.

When human rights activists and psychiatrists have invoked the concept of paternalism, they have been partly drawing on discussions in Western political theory and medical ethics about paternalism—that is, whether and when other people, institutions, or the state is justified in interfering with a person's liberty to promote that person's interests (Buchanan 1978; Dworkin 1972; New 1999). Situated in liberal democracies, these discussions all prioritize individual autonomy. This has also been valorized, or at least gestured toward, in China's mental health legislative debates, and it is why patient autonomy has been established as a principle of the MHL. At the same time, Chinese activists and psychiatrists have invoked other paternalistic traditions, including Confucian ideas of paternal authority, filial piety, and family-state isomorphism, as well as the socialist tradition of encouraging or even requiring people to work for, depend on, and develop a paternal identification with the state in exchange for promises of protection, provision, and prosperity (Steinmüller 2015; Verdery 1996). Not all of these traditions endorse individual autonomy, but they each involve an authority structure in which one party decides on what is good for another party and seeks to bring it about in action (Barnett 2017).

In this book, I take an interpretive approach to examine how people define, enact, and value autonomy in practice and what other shapes of subjectivity they envision. In contemporary China, forces of marketization, privatization, and global capital are entangled with "the lingering effects of socialist institutions and practices" (Zhang 2001, 179). Thus, I also take a historical, ideological, and structural approach to ask to what extent the promises of state paternalism are upheld, who actually carries the responsibility for being paternal, and what it looks like to practice paternalism in everyday life. While most existing studies have ignored the gendered dimension in the implementation of paternalism,[13] I explore how women or other vulnerable individuals, as supposed agents of paternalism, might enact or alter it.

As this book will reveal, although drafters of the MHL acknowledged the idea of patient autonomy, they were concerned with the damages it might bring to patients and society, which had presumably happened in capitalist countries. Therefore, they framed the widespread use of involuntary psychiatric interventions in China as a perk of socialism (chapter 1). Indeed, as these interventions continue to dominate the landscape of mental health care, to many people, freedom from them appears to be indicative of neglect (chapter 5). Note that the subject of state paternalism that the drafters of the MHL envisioned was no longer the socialist proletariat but a carrier of pathology and risk needing to be managed. Unable to ensure the state's financial commitment, they relegated the responsibilities of paternalistic action to patients' families. Chapters 2 and 4 show how, outside of the legislative debates, hospital psychiatry and community mental health practices have been expecting and inculcating families to be intimate authorities devoted to risk management, powerful enough to summon patients' compliance. Nevertheless, because the primary caregivers are typically ageing parents or other female relatives, they are often unable and unwilling to act paternalistically as expected. Instead, they may engage in maternal, supplemental practices to address patients'—and their own—vulnerabilities. In addition to these quiet, spontaneous disruptions, chapter 6 shows some caregivers' conscious struggles for what I call "paternalistic citizenship": they demand that the state not only recognize their contribution to managing risk and maintaining public order but also live up to its promises and perform proper paternal *guan* itself—by looking after its vulnerable citizens and repairing any damage wrought by marketization.

Attention to these keywords helps unearth the conditions, operations, and repercussions of biopolitical paternalism. In the neoliberal, postwelfare world, many people long for a paternalistic state (Street 2012) while fearing its potential overreach (Aretxaga 2003), having to rely on the family's warmth but worrying about its precarity and restrictions. My study provides an analytic for teasing out complexities and imagining new possibilities in the logics and practices of governance. Back to mental health, it also allows us to explicate the hopes and fears of people who experience madness and psychiatry to consider whether total control or abstract freedom is really what they need, and it explores how their needs can be addressed through new forms of social policies and public responsibilities. Because these keywords travel widely while undergoing constant reconfiguration and contestation, an ethnographic methodology that traces their circulation in different realms and that engages with different stakeholders is warranted.

Methodological Journey

Encountering Psychiatry and the Family

The journey that led me to the intersection of madness, family, and psychiatry was tortuous. In hindsight, it was a practice of what Donna Haraway (1991) called "situated knowledges," enabled by many chance encounters that revealed people's "contestation, deconstruction, [and] passionate construction" (191) of patienthood and care. It also required much "engaged, accountable [re-]positioning" (196) on my end to foster "webbed connections . . . and hope of [the] transformation of systems of knowledge and ways of seeing" (191–92).

My first encounter with psychiatry was during my undergraduate years in Beijing as a psychology major. In a psychopathology class, students were asked to interview inpatients in a major psychiatric hospital to assess their symptomatic manifestations. The patient to whom I was assigned was a woman who had been hospitalized by her family members for schizophrenia for eleven years. I could easily follow the teacher's instructions and fit the woman's words into the diagnostic manual. Yet I was struck by her despair over her prolonged seclusion and by the entanglements between her illness experience and her troubled family life, such as her stigmatizing childhood experience living with a father who had also been diagnosed with schizophrenia. Since then, I have been intrigued by the psychiatric institution and fascinated by the sociocultural underpinnings of illness experiences. It was this fascination that led me to travel halfway around the world to study cultural and medical anthropology in the United States.

In the summers of 2008 and 2009, I began conducting fieldwork at the Benevolence Hospital, which had 168 licensed psychiatrists, 469 nurses, and

1,920 beds (as of 2009). A flagship psychiatric hospital in the city of Nanhua and even throughout Southern China, it allowed me to observe and analyze Chinese psychiatry in an optimal form. Meanwhile, the crowded space and the staff's heavy caseload at Benevolence resembled most other psychiatric hospitals in China. My initial access to Benevolence was facilitated by a family friend and by my bachelor's degree in psychology from a prestigious university. Although the hospital was biomedically oriented, its administrators and doctors saw my knowledge as potentially beneficial to the inpatients. I was stationed on the adult psychiatry wards, which primarily housed people diagnosed with schizophrenia and other psychotic disorders along with some individuals diagnosed with bipolar disorder or other mental illnesses. Every day, I joined the staff for morning meetings and ward rounds and observed psychiatrists as they wrote medical records or met with families in the office. When little was happening in the office, I went inside the locked ward to chat with patients. Most of them liked talking with me, because few staff members had the interest or time to listen to their concerns.

At the time, my interest was in how doctors, patients, and families experienced schizophrenia and how their explanations of the illness were shaped by various cultural knowledges (Ma 2012). During fieldwork, I could not help but realize that most patients on the wards had been forcibly or deceptively hospitalized by their family members and that most were resentful of that experience. Some people complained to me that their "symptoms" had been fabricated by their family members. Others might not question their diagnoses but were afraid of being left in the ward by their family members forever. Listening to their sighs and cries, it was hard for me to look the other way or make cultural generalizations that were disengaged from their struggles.

Gradually, my focus turned to families' involvement in psychiatric care. I returned to Benevolence's adult psychiatry wards and visited its outpatient clinic for brief follow-ups over the subsequent summers and for eighteen months during 2013–2014. Through interviews and observation, I examined why people turned to psychiatry for help, what it meant for family members to care for patients, on what ground they claimed the authority, knowledge, and responsibility to do so, and how such acts were perceived. I also observed the power relations in these practices, such as whose voice had been silenced, whose suffering had gone unrecognized, and the life options and relationships that had either been enabled or thwarted. To understand how individuals' views on ethical practices had been shaped by psychiatry, I observed how doctors solicited patients' illness histories from their family members, how doctors taught patients the nature of their illnesses and the importance of medical treatment, and how family members were inculcated with ways to manage patients. I also examined patients' and family members' reception to, and challenges of, these psychiatric instructions.

Charting the Mental Health Landscape

My new interest in families required me to chart a broader landscape of institutions and agencies involved in serving, monitoring, and challenging families' involvement in psychiatric care. Fortunately, the mental health infrastructure in Nanhua and its province was more established and comprehensive than that of many other parts of China. Since 2004, and especially after 2010, the National Ministry of Health has rolled out a community mental health program across China, which regards family caregivers as crucial allies in the management of people diagnosed with SMIS. Benevolence's staff kindly introduced me to several community mental health practitioners in both urban and rural areas of the city. I was able to observe their everyday work—especially visits to patients' homes—in the summers of 2010 and 2011 and then again during 2013–2014. I paid attention to how these practitioners obtained information about patients' illnesses and risk of violence from caregivers, their discussions with caregivers about the nature of the illness and proper family care, as well as any interventions the practitioners undertook for patients or their families.

Moreover, Nanhua had one of the earliest, and still leading, mental health social work agencies in China called the BeWell Family Resource Center. Built and mainly funded by the municipal government, its founding mission was to serve the family members of people recovering from SMIS and to encourage them to become resources for each other. Typical services included weekly informational meetings, support groups, and individual casework. As of 2014, the center had a registered clientele of over 1,000 caregivers, among whom about 100 were regular participants. Besides serving family members, the center had also developed vocational training classes and a sheltered workshop, at which persons recovering from SMIS could receive vocational training and low-wage employment opportunities. During my long-term fieldwork in 2013–2014, I spent much time at BeWell, participating in its activities as a researcher and volunteer, and observing how notions of family, mental illness, and care were imparted, discussed, and challenged. I also accompanied family members and patients outside the center as they navigated health care and welfare resources, helped each other with various life difficulties, or simply had fun together. From January to May 2014, I lived in the city's largest public housing community, whose residents included over 300 people with psychiatric disabilities and their family members. BeWell had established a branch there to serve them. This "deep hanging out" (Rosaldo 1994) gave me further insight into people's everyday lives, which were partially connected to, but not subsumed by, BeWell or other institutions.

In examining these pioneering institutions in Nanhua, I was less concerned with representing "China" as a whole. After all, it is hard for any situated ethnographic study to do so given the country's internal diversities. Instead, I was interested in exploring potentialities—that is, how new trends in the mental health field might reinforce, destabilize, or remake the meaning of patient care and the family's role in it, as configured by the psychiatric hospital. Meanwhile, over the years, to gain a more balanced view of different socioeconomic conditions, I visited various hospitals, community mental health teams, and (where they existed) social work/rehabilitation centers in other parts of China, from Beijing and Shanghai to provincial capitals like Kunming and to small cities and rural counties in Southern China. My visits ranged from half-day tours for interviews with administrators or senior staff to days or even weeks of observation. This book will draw on these visits to supplement my data from Nanhua.

The present is not just oriented toward the future but also situated in the past. As such, we need to understand how the family has been variably configured since the late 1890s, how these configurations have been shaped by sociopolitical changes and developments in psychiatric expertise, and how they have become discursive and institutional threads that weave into the present. To do so, I consulted archival materials on Chinese psychiatry at Yale Divinity School, the Shanghai Library Bibliotheca Zi-Ka-Wei, and the Needham Research Institute in the United Kingdom. Benevolence's institutional history was not well preserved, but I still managed to learn bits and pieces by reading the generations of books and hospital publications in its library and by checking files on it in Nanhua's municipal archives.

Tracking the Mental Health Law

Just as I was drawn to studying families' controversial involvement in psychiatry, I noticed news articles about people wrongfully diagnosed with mental illness and hospitalized. Some articles also mentioned the protracted course of establishing national mental health legislation. Following this lead,

I traveled around China to interview nationally leading psychiatrists who had been involved in drafting the legislation. Interview topics included the family's role in inpatient and community care as set out in the drafts and as perceived by those psychiatrists; the state's responsibilities for patient care and management; and how those experts responded to public controversy surrounding involuntary hospitalization and coercive treatment initiated by families or other agents.

In 2011, I met with staffers of a Shenzhen-based organization called the Equity and Justice Initiative (EJI).[14] As the only organization in Mainland China dedicated to advocating for the rights of psychiatric patients, the EJI had collected cases of psychiatric abuse, connected self-proclaimed victims to legal support, published reports for domestic and international readers, and engaged in public debates with psychiatrists on the mental health legal reform. When conducting fieldwork in Nanhua, I often visited Shenzhen and elsewhere to participate in workshops organized by the EJI. I also traveled with its staff to national and international conferences on the mental health legal reform and on disability rights. Through these interactions, I became familiar with the ideas of EJI staff on the proper relationship between mental illness, family guardianship, and human rights, as well as their plans, strategies, and the obstacles they encountered in promoting patient autonomy. In addition to these face-to-face conversations with key parties, I also tracked public discussions around the mental health legislation as they appeared in the media.

Now that the MHL has come into effect, one needs to examine its interpretation, implementation, and impact in practice. My prolonged fieldwork, spanning from 2008 to 2014, provided an ideal time window to assess both change and continuity in the mental health field. As sociolegal scholars have noted, while the law can transform society and shape people's consciousness, its interpretation is also shaped by culturally and historically embedded social relations (Yngvesson 1988). Moreover, in organizational practices and informal settings, the law is activated far more often than in the courts. It is the decisions made and routines established in these situations that effectively become the law that people implement (Sarat and Kearns 1995). Therefore, besides tracing the few formal legal proceedings that invoked the MHL, I also observed how grassroots health-care professionals, government officials, family members, and patients interpreted and enacted the law; how they invoked it to discuss care and management as well as rights and responsibilities; and what institutional and socioeconomic conditions shaped these interpretations. Of special interest were patient admission and discharge procedures, the two most controversial areas of psychiatric practice as reflected in the legislative debates.

Building Better Worlds

Mental health in China is a contested field, because different parties often hold diametrically opposed views about proper arrangements for patients. Especially during the legislative debates, psychiatrists/policymakers and human rights activists would excoriate each other, and each side saw itself as the righteous spokesperson of both patients and the public. It was tricky for me to navigate between them: for instance, knowing that I was interested in studying families' involvement in hospitalization, some senior psychiatrists in a renowned hospital saw me as a human rights activist unable to understand their position, or worse still, as an American spy intent on digging up dirt on China. As a result, they rejected my application to conduct part of my research in their institution. Therefore, when conducting fieldwork, I had to be careful not to identify myself with any one group, lest it prevent me from accessing others.

Nevertheless, as I gradually earned the trust of my interlocutors, and as I better understood their visions and omissions, I started facilitating dialogues between different parties. For example, the EJI once invited me to its workshop on deinstitutionalization. From previous interactions, I knew that because of its focus on individual autonomy, its advocacy overlooked individuals' experiences of vulnerability and their needs for care. Therefore, instead of attending the workshop alone, I brought along more than thirty interested patients and caregivers. They spoke about their horrific experiences with various institutions and the need for legal oversight. Instead of advocating for complete deinstitutionalization, however, many discussed ways institutions should be improved, alternative services that could be provided, and care networks that might be built beyond one's immediate relatives. Their powerful words shook both the EJI staff and me. Seeing how thoughtful their loved ones were also caused some caregivers present to rethink their equation of mental illness with inability. For another example, as the biomedical model and psychiatric hospitals dominated the mental health field, oftentimes patients and families were unaware of other health or social services available. As a person who had the privilege of visiting different sites and organizations, I often found myself assuming the role of a social worker, connecting my interlocutors to organizations and resources that might benefit them.

Thus, rather than simply studying a preexisting "field," the fieldwork that constitutes this book contains efforts from my various interlocutors and myself to build helpful connections and better worlds together. By charting convergences and ruptures in family care and professional services, I hope this book generates more dialogue, understanding, and collaborative endeavors among people and entities concerned with mental health services, both within and beyond China. As such, it is an exercise of "a *committed and engaged* anthropology" (Forman 1995, 3).

Chapter Organization

A brief roadmap may help readers navigate the complex research journey condensed in this book. As I mentioned, chapter 1 traces how the hospital-family circuit has come to dominate mental health care for persons diagnosed with SMIs in reform-era China. Against this backdrop, it examines how activists and psychiatrists have struggled to define patient rights along with the meaning and legitimacy of paternalism in mental health legislative debates. In the next three chapters, I employ a slightly anachronistic approach and explore family practices in relation to institutions and community agents before the MHL to contrast the abstract legal language with the concrete ways paternalism and the related idea of *guan* have been inculcated, enacted, or resisted. Chapter 2 shows how everyday hospital practices translate people's experiences of chaos into symptoms of a mental disorder, turning family members' desire for *guan* into lifelong responsibility for risk management. Chapter 3 explores how this vision of risk and responsibility reworks family relations, dissolving certain ties while isolating others. Chapter 4 examines how the new national community mental health program, especially its agenda of preventing patients' risks of violence, further mobilizes and shapes family life and how family members engage in practices that simultaneously disrupt and supplement this agenda. In chapters 3 and 4, I highlight how the relational practices of female and feminized caregivers differ from, and supplement, the paternalism practiced by male family members or mandated by state programs.

Chapter 5 returns (or moves forward again) to the MHL and examines its implementation, focusing on how the interplay between interpretations of risk (now the sole criterion for involuntary hospitalization), institutional arrangements, and people's sense of responsibility influences hospital admission and discharge processes. Chapter 6 turns to the collective actions and narrations of family caregivers, especially how they deploy the state's paternalistic promises to stake citizenship claims, individually or together. Finally, the conclusion discusses resonances of biopolitical paternalism in other aspects of contemporary Chinese life, its recent transformations during the COVID-19 pandemic, and its implications for conceptualizing governance and care throughout the world. I also revisit what happened to Xu Wei after the trial and imagine how we could help people like him by disrupting the harm caused by biopolitical paternalism.

1

CONSTRUCTING FAMILIES,
CONTESTING PATERNALISMS

On a cold winter day in 2013, Chen Dan,[1] a female engineer in her early thirties, met with me over a hot-pot dinner in Beijing. Ten days before, she had lost a case in which she had sued a psychiatric hospital for violating her rights to personal freedom. On June 5, 2012, four male strangers broke into Chen's apartment in Beijing. They were followed by her parents, who, according to her, hated her boyfriend and wanted her back home in Northeast China. The strangers snatched her from her boyfriend, put her in a van, and drove her to the hospital. At the outpatient clinic, a doctor met with her parents. After a brief conversation with them, he wrote a diagnosis of "agitation" on Chen's medical records. Meanwhile, watched by one of the strangers in the hallway, Chen furtively texted her friends for help. A moment later, she found herself in a locked inpatient ward, her cell phone confiscated by a nurse.

Initially scared, Chen quickly collected her thoughts. She told doctors on the ward about her estranged relationship with her parents, insisted that she was not sick, and threatened to sue the hospital if she was not released immediately. Alerted, psychiatrists of various ranks came to question her, and they finally diagnosed her as having "recurrent depressive disorder, remission stage" because her parents had said that she had felt unhappy about a previous breakup and had once sought counseling. Against her parents' objection, the hospital released her to her boyfriend at the end of the third day, claiming that she was "in remission" and thus did not need hospitalization.

Upon her release, Chen contacted Huang Xuetao, a prominent human rights lawyer and activist on mental health issues. Huang quickly summoned the press, which attacked the hospital for wrongfully committing the innocent, "normal," and capable young woman—a process they called "being mentally illed" (被精神病/*bei jingshenbing*; Xi 2013)—thereby violating her right to autonomy. In response, the hospital held a press conference with the theme "Being mentally illed is not as simple as you think." At the conference, the hospital staff reported Chen's illness history as it had been collected from her parents, including her "suicidal behavior" and "paranoid" view that her parents would harm her. They argued that the decision to hospitalize Chen had adhered to the Beijing Mental Health Regulation's stipulation on medical protection hospitalization, which allowed guardians to hospitalize people diagnosed with SMIs against their will and aimed to protect the patient's right to health (Wang and Li 2012).

Shortly after the press conference, Chen filed suit against the hospital. In court, Chen's attorney argued that the Beijing Regulation was inapplicable because depression did not count as an SMI under the law and that as an adult with full legal capacity, she should not be placed under her parents' guardianship. Nevertheless, the court ruled in favor of the defense, saying that if Chen's parents had provided inaccurate information to the hospital, then they, not the hospital, should be responsible for any violation of rights. It also decreed that although the doctors had not diagnosed Chen with an SMI, the "complexity and variability" entailed in how mental illness could manifest justified the inpatient observation (Chen 2013).

When we met, Chen complained about not just the hospital and the court but also her oppressive family. She saw her parents as paranoid, antisocial, and obsessed with her: they thought all her friends, including her boyfriend, intended to harm her, and they were concerned that life in the city was corrupting her. She often had to move to escape their control, but she still could not avoid being kidnapped and taken to the hospital. According to Chen, Chinese parents often exert such domination while claiming that it is for their children's own good. To cure this pathological culture, she argued, "mental health regulations should be concerned with the sick parents, not the bullied children." As Chen saw it, the Chinese legal system tends to give parents (and other senior family members) immunity, regardless of the injuries they inflict, entrenching a culture of paternalistic control that prevails in the family and even the state. Chen said: "State paternalism is like that of the family. If you dare to oppose the state, even if the state is wrong, it will deprive you of rights, because it wants to control you. The same goes for the family. Parents may be wrong, but they want to control you, because they are the ones in power."

Constructing, Debating, and Scaling Paternalism in Chinese Psychiatry

As mentioned in the introduction, most psychiatric inpatients in China were hospitalized against their will by their family members before the MHL. Cases like Chen's both reflected and challenged this common practice, and they helped propel the final passage of the MHL, the drafting of which had begun as early as 1985. In the mental health legislative debates, human rights activists, ex-patients, and allied journalists used terms such as *being mentally illed* to frame involuntary hospitalization as a violation of an individual's right to autonomy, whereas psychiatrists framed it as a measure to protect patients' right to health. Both sides saw such interventions as undergirded by paternalism, though they defined and evaluated it in opposite ways: while activists defined paternalism negatively as oppressive control in the name of love, psychiatrists saw it positively as care for the vulnerable and the less knowledgeable. As the product of these debates, the MHL affirms patient autonomy and the voluntary principle of hospitalization; at the same time, it upholds families' guardianship of patients and stipulates a series of rights and responsibilities regarding patient treatment, management, and provision.

Why did both the activists' and the psychiatrists' views make it into the MHL? How does the law embrace the seemingly contradictory principles of patient autonomy and family guardianship? This chapter investigates these puzzles by examining not just the legislative debates but also the historically sedimented landscape of mental health care in China on which different parties have staked their claims, especially the hospital-family circuit that captured Chen Dan and many others diagnosed with mental illness. As suggested in the introduction, the family is not just a site of care and the relational dynamics that come with it. It is also an ideological and institutional construct with which people imagine and shape the meaning of the good life, the pathway to achieve it, and the authority, expertise, and responsibilities involved in doing so. For instance, at the turn of the twentieth century, medical missionaries justified the establishment of asylums as a liberatory project by portraying Chinese families as oppressive patriarchies emblematic of a backward culture and society. In the first half of this chapter, I will continue to trace the changing ideas around the family in the People's Republic: whereas the Maoist regime downplayed the role of individual families in social reproduction but fashioned itself as a parent state that cared and provided for its people, public discourses in the market reform era have naturalized the family as an essential space of intimacy and nurturance. These ideas were conditioned by health and social policies of their times, and they in turn shored up different logics and operations of mental health care.

As such, psychiatric discourses and social policies in different eras have variably constructed individual households or the state as paternalistic, positively or negatively, in resemblance or contrast to each other. Building on these legacies, the idea of paternalism in contemporary China is not only multivalent but also scalable. That is, people can expand or contract the scope of its signification without rethinking its basic elements (Tsing 2012). Indeed, as I will show in the second half of this chapter, it was by using historical resources explicitly and implicitly to define and scale paternalism that stakeholders debated the ethics of mental health practices and the content of the MHL. For example, in the opening vignette, Chen Dan complained about paternalism in families as well as the state which had enabled it. She also complained about how state paternalism resembled the paternalism in families. Meanwhile, the psychiatrists who had drafted the law defended involuntary hospitalization as a manifestation of state paternalism while reinforcing individual families' authority to act paternalistically. As they scaled paternalism, these stakeholders also scaled up and down issues of psychiatric abuse to lay claims over the subjects and rights at stake. That is, they sorted, grouped, categorized, and compared the phenomena pertaining to mental health practices "in terms of relative degrees of elevation and centrality" (Carr and Lempert 2016, 3) to argue over what problem the law should address and how.

In the end, the intricate discursive game of scaling led to a compromise in the MHL: whereas struggles about paternalism's desirability were concentrated on the state level, the responsibility of enacting or rejecting it in practice was left to the family. Scholars have noted that by moving a phenomenon across scales, one can locate it in a particular "historical timespace" (Blommaert 2007) in relation to a vision of the geopolitical order (Klinke 2013). By examining how paternalism has been constructed on different scales and how it has been scaled in the legislative debates, we can explicate the trajectory of social development that stakeholders envisioned for China as well as the forms of life and relations that it elevated, took for granted, or erased.

*State Paternalism and Community
Mobilization during the Maoist Era*

If missionary psychiatrists and their Republican successors had problematized the Chinese family as a patriarchy to critique, utilize, or intervene into, then the Maoist state had constructed itself—positively—as what scholars have called a "public patriarchy," "parent state," or "state paternalism" (Stacey 1983; Walder 1988). It did so by downplaying the role of individual families, organizing people into collectives such as urban work units and rural communes, providing them with broader and more equal access to resources, and directly portraying Mao as the father of the country-family (Steinmüller 2015). As a manifestation of this state paternalism, almost everyone—including nonworking dependents—was covered by urban labor insurance or the rural cooperative medical system, so their medical expenses were minimal (Duckett 2012).

Psychiatry resumed its development as China recovered from years of war. By the mid-1950s, the country had 46 mental hospitals and clinics, 11,000 beds, 400 psychiatrists, and 4,600 mental health workers, psychologists, and nurses—16–20 times the number in 1949. Treatment during this period included psychopharmaceuticals such as chlorpromazine and lithium, insulin, electroshock therapy (which was later banned during the Cultural Revolution), and traditional Chinese medical techniques such as herbs, acupuncture, and moxibustion. Influenced by Maoist thought, psychiatrists in this era tended to see mental illness as a harmful aftermath of the bourgeois society or obsession with the bourgeois worldview; thus, they used political education, work therapy, and cultural activities to rid patients of these harmful influences and to help reintegrate them into the proletariat revolution (Kao 1979).

In the 1960s and 1970s, as Mao sought to radically deinstitutionalize politics and expand grassroots mobilization, hospital psychiatry gave way to community care. Psychiatrists spent years in villages training barefoot doctors—individuals who received rudimentary training to treat common diseases and conduct basic public health work while also working their day jobs—or other grassroots medical personnel, helping them establish mental health stations to deliver accessible treatment. Many cities also saw the establishment of community guardianship networks, in which retirees, neighbors, and street-level officials joined forces to give patients and their families material and emotional support (Pearson 1995; Phillips 1998). As such, in the Maoist era, families were far from the sole caregivers, nor were hospitals the only venues for treatment. While these arrangements would change dramatically, the idea of the state taking an active, paternalistic role in envisioning and providing mental health care would continue to shape the perspective of the seasoned psychiatrists who went on to frame the MHL.

Market Reform, Family Nurturance, and Psychiatric Institutionalization

In the market reform era, the individual family was reconfigured as the default symbolic and material source of life. In 1981, the Central government started promoting the household contract responsibility system in rural areas, which allowed household members to band together as a production unit to earn profits. Thereby, the communes and the rural cooperative medical system they had run gradually dissolved. In urban areas, state-owned enterprises (SOEs) began undergoing restructuring in the mid-1980s and went into bankruptcy en masse in the 1990s. The labor health insurance at the time did not cover people who were unemployed or who had begun working in the private sector. Even for those who had remained in SOEs, health-care coverage typically became much more limited and excluded dependents. As a result, from 1993 to 2003, only 30 percent of the population was covered by any medical insurance, and the proportion of out-of-pocket expenses to overall health-care spending rose from 20 percent in 1978 to 61 percent in 2000 (Duckett 2012). Pressured by outcry against the broken safety net, the state has been rebuilding and expanding the public insurance systems since 2002 (Blumenthal and Hsiao 2005). Yet unemployed persons typically need to pay substantial premiums to opt in, and their coverage is less extensive than that of employed persons. The public health insurance also only covers a limited catalogue of treatment and medications. As such, the health-care expenses of the unemployed, insured or not, fall heavily on their families.

In the Maoist era, the Ministry of the Interior (later the Ministry of Civil Affairs) built a system of psychiatric hospitals to provide free treatment to people with mental illnesses who had no home, support, or means of livelihood (Pearson 1995). At its peak, this system housed over 20 percent of China's psychiatric beds—most of the other beds were in psychiatric hospitals supervised by the Ministry of Health. The rest were general or psychiatric hospitals for persons who had been convicted of crimes and were supervised by the Ministry of Public Security (Phillips 1998). In 1987, the Ministry of Civil Affairs ordered its hospitals to change their mission and develop self-paid care instead. Vice Minister Zhang Dejiang, who would later become one of China's highest-ranking leaders, explained the change this way: "With the increase in living standards of the people and the continuous development of society there are fewer and fewer mental patients who have no family to go to, no financial resources and no supportive network. There are more and more who are doing nothing productive for society but who do have family support" (Pearson 1995, 75).

This statement measured an individual's value against the labor productivity expected by the market, viewed the provision for the supposedly valueless psychiatric patients as a natural task of their families, and assumed that families were available to (and desirable for) almost everyone. Although the psychiatric hospitals run by the Ministry of Civil Affairs were not prevalent throughout China, this statement indicated a sweeping change in this era. For instance, while the 1950 Marriage Law only stated in a general sense that parents should provide for their children (Government Administration Council of the Central People's Government 1950, Article 13), its 1980 revisions explicitly stipulated that parents should provide for adult children who could not live independently (National People's Congress 1980, Article 21). Taken together, these discursive and institutional arrangements have made the family a basic unit of production, reproduction, and survival in the reform era.

In this era, the field of psychiatry has also undergone a sea change. As the Chinese state has deviated from the idea of grassroots mobilization, turning instead to elite science and the globalization that it symbolizes (Greenhalgh 2020), barefoot doctors and primary health workers have been dismissed as unprofessional or unable to provide advanced treatment. Concurrently, psychiatrists have returned to the center stage, and this time their approach is resolutely biomedical: their diagnoses are shaped by American and international diagnostic standards (Lee 2001), and they view mental illness as resulting from neurochemical imbalances. Most psychiatrists would sneer at the idea that sociopolitical processes might have any role in causing or treating mental illness (Achtenberg 1983). They also refuse to understand mental illness from the perspective of traditional Chinese medicine, although they might follow patients, or families' requests to use it to ameliorate psychopharmaceutical side effects (Lin and Ma 2023; Ma 2012). Note that while the practice and teaching of psychotherapy was restored in the 1980s and has boomed in the twenty-first century (Huang 2015; J. Yang 2015; Zhang 2020), it is not regarded as appropriate for people with SMIs in mainstream Chinese psychiatry.

Hand in hand with the professionalization and biomedicalization of psychiatry has been the rise of large institutions. Since the 1980s, leading psychiatrists have vocally lamented China's shortage of hospital-based mental health services and called for their expansion (Pearson 1995), often ignoring the existing rich community practices. This was understandable in the sense that as local governments became increasingly focused on economic growth, they defunded and privatized community clinics, destroying the primary health system and people's faith in it. At any rate, partly thanks to the advocacy, from 1978 to 2009, the number of psychiatric hospitals in China increased from 219 to 637, the number of psychiatric beds increased from 42,000 to 191,000, and the number of psychiatrists increased from 3,128 to 18,800 (Li et al. 2012). Most of these psychiatrists and beds are concentrated in specialized psychiatric hospitals rather than general hospitals.

Note, however, that government support accounts for less than 30 percent of the income of so-called public hospitals (Gong, Feng, and Wang 2005). Most of this financial support goes to infrastructural development, equipment purchases, and hospital staffs' base salaries. The hospitals themselves are responsible for everyday expenses and the staff's bonuses, and they in turn exert financial pressure on departments and individual physicians. Because of the kickbacks routinely handed out by pharmaceutical and medical device companies, physicians often prescribe expensive drugs and procedures, many of which are not covered by public health insurance.[2] In psychiatric hospitals, physicians also tend to promote inpatient treatment, for it allows them to not only closely monitor patients but also to prescribe a wide variety of medications and tests, as well as elective services and therapies. During my fieldwork in 2008–2014, the standard course of inpatient treatment recommended by psychiatrists at Benevolence lasted for three months, and the cost was CNY 6,000–10,000 per month (other less renowned hospitals charged slightly less, but all were above CNY 4,000), whereas the average annual income for residents in Nanhua was slightly under CNY 6,000. Because many people diagnosed with SMIs are unemployed, paying for these bills or securing public resources becomes a responsibility for, and a strain on, their families.

Insight, Involuntary Admission, and the
Hospital-Family Circuit

Families are not just central to financing psychiatric hospitalization but also to the process of knowledge production and decision-making. From the psychiatrists' perspective, many people with SMIs lack insight (自知力/*zizhili*), or "the ability to realize, understand, and describe one's abnormal mental status and pathological behavior" (Shanghai Municipal People's Congress 2001, Article 47). This reflects a larger disorder of the self as a bounded, coherent, agentive, and introspective entity. The self-disorder is a key feature of SMIS, and it manifests in symptoms such as delusion, hallucinations, and disorganized behavior (Ma 2012). Whereas traditional Chinese medicine saw madness as a phenomenon readily recognizable by others, psychiatry's emphasis on the self makes the narration of personal experience crucial for diagnosis; it also deems the self-report from the person without insight to be unreliable. Who, then, is in the position to account for the person's changing experience? Many psychiatrists turn to family members, who are supposed to have intimate knowledge about the person. Especially before the MHL, psychiatric textbooks often instructed doctors to collect illness histories from family members, ideally without the patient's knowledge, to avoid any confrontation (Zhao 2008). We saw this at work in Chen Dan's hospital admission.

From the psychiatric perspective, the lack of insight also requires others—that is, family members—to receive medical information and make treatment decisions for the person. A survey in the early 2000s showed that most psychiatric inpatients had been hospitalized against their will, typically by their family members (Pan, Xie, and Zheng 2003). These inpatients would not be discharged unless the parties who had committed them came to pick them up, because hospitals wanted to avoid any liability and ensure that the bills were paid (Huang, Liu, and Liu 2010). Therefore, the fact that Chen Dan was released to her boyfriend and not her parents was unusual, indicating how much pressure the hospital was under. Between 2002 and 2012, seven cities in China, including Shanghai, Beijing, and Shenzhen, issued municipal mental health regulations. They all declared that "patients or family members" had the right to make informed consent to treatment. They also all stipulated that family members could hospitalize patients who had no insight and thus no "capacity for civil conduct" (Chen 2023, 71), with several regulations using the term *medical protection hospitalization* to describe this procedure: "A certified psychiatrist's duty is only to advise that the patient be admitted. The patient's family member or guardian has the right to decide whether to accept the advice or not, and when to finish or withdraw from the hospitalization and treatment" (Shao et al. 2010, 5). As the word *protection* suggests, the regulations framed the commitment procedure in terms of beneficence, a basic medical ethics principle, for it would supposedly bring patients the treatment they needed and improve their well-being as defined by psychiatry, even against their objections.

Of course, in reform-era China, family members also play a huge role in making decisions about other medical practices. For instance, the 1999 Medical Practitioners Law used the phrase *patients or family members* when referring to informed consent; the 2010 Tort Law clarified that medical staff should seek informed consent from the patient, but when that is inappropriate—often read as including situations like mental illness and cancer—they should seek informed consent from the patient's close relatives (Du and Feng 2017). These laws and customs might have shaped mental health practices and regulations, but mental illness also provided an occasion for lawmakers to articulate the conditions of substitute decision-making. Beyond China, some countries, such as Japan and Mexico, also largely rely on families to commit persons to psychiatric hospitals. Yet in these countries, hospitalization is either viewed as a last resort and a form of abandonment for a few desperate families (Reyes-Foster 2018), or it is in decline with rising deinstitutionalization and independent living movements (Nakamura 2013). In contrast, as this book will clarify, hospitalization in China is expanding and being promoted as a good that caring families should want for their loved ones with mental illness.

In short, in the market reform era, families, instead of the state, have become the agents of paternalism. They assume heavy responsibilities for caring for people diagnosed with smis and the primary authority of imposing certain forms of care, especially hospitalization and psychopharmaceutical treatment. This position results from the retreat of public welfare; the naturalization of family nurturance and intimate knowledge; the biomedicalization, institutionalization, and commercialization of health care; and the view of a person with smi as a disordered self that is valueless until cured by psychiatry. Through this configuration, a hospital-family circuit of mental health care emerges, where the patient is shuffled between the home and the hospital and where the family becomes the closest ally and primary consumer of psychiatry.[3]

Debating Paternalism and Rights in Mental Health Legislation

China's mental health legislative process began in the early reform era. In 1985, as part of a government-wide effort to modernize the country's legal system, the Ministry of Health (MoH) commissioned Dr. Liu Xiehe, a forensic psychiatrist in Sichuan, to lead the drafting of a national mental health law. As Dr. Liu recalled in my interview, he promptly summoned help from his colleagues, consulted experts from the World Health Organization (WHO), and solicited opinions on the task from relevant government sectors. Nevertheless, the drafts he submitted to the MoH in the 1990s strangely sank into oblivion. In 1999, the MoH convened younger psychiatrists to revive the drafting process (Phillips et al. 2013), and they helped pass the aforementioned seven pieces of municipal mental health legislation as test runs for the national law. These regulations largely endorsed the de facto practice of involuntary hospitalization and families' primary authority over it. Outside the small group of drafting psychiatrists and government officials, few knew of the legislating efforts. It was not until the mid-2000s, when ex-patients and human rights activists started to condemn involuntary hospitalization on media, that the public became aware of issues pertaining to psychiatry and law. In 2009, the Legislative Affairs Office of the State Council took over the law's drafting from the MoH, and in 2012, it passed the baton to the Standing Committee of the National People's Congress, China's paramount legislative organ (Ding 2014). (Psychiatrists were still closely consulted in these processes.) In October 2012, the MHL was finally passed, and it came into effect in May 2013. As we will see below, it was by strategically framing and scaling the issue of involuntary hospitalization that activists succeeded in drawing widespread attention and setting the terms of the legislation.

Human Rights Campaigns and Challenges
against Paternalism

In 2006, lawyer Huang Xuetao became involved in challenging the hospitalization of a thirty-year-old woman named Zou Yijun. Zou had recently lost her father and gotten divorced. Her father had bequeathed a house to her, and the divorce had brought her a large settlement. A Buddhist devotee, she wanted to use the money for a religious study tour, but her mother and brother wanted to rent out the house and use her settlement money for a downpayment on a new apartment. As their fight progressed, Zou felt unsafe and gave her friend Huang Xuetao—then a corporate lawyer—power of attorney, authorizing Huang to exercise her civil rights on her behalf if she lost her freedom. In a family visit to her father's grave, Zou was taken away by male assailants, tranquilized, and sent to a psychiatric hospital. There, she was registered under a pseudonym and diagnosed with bipolar disorder. To rescue Zou, Huang called the police and forced the hospital to acknowledge her admission. Then she gathered a crowd of journalists in front of the hospital to demand a meeting between the two of them. The hospital staff initially refused the request, claiming that a person with mental illness did not have the legal capacity to seek representation, but they ultimately gave in to the media pressure and released Zou.

After this incident, Huang began advocating for psychiatric patients' rights, and she later established a nongovernmental organization called the Equity and Justice Initiative (EJI). Working with ex-patients and allies, they endeavored to provoke, frame, and guide public discussion about mental health legislation. Initially, they called psychiatric hospitals "prisons by contract" (契约监狱/*qiyue jianyu*): because the hospitals had to finance themselves, they would do anything to get paid, even locking people up without legal grounds (Zhou 2009). Because the families were usually the payers, both the hospitals and the paternalistic culture of the families were in need of reform. Or as Zou Yijun stated in a televised interview, "We cannot deprive citizens of all their rights and freedom in the name of love" (Anonymous 2009). The phrase *prisons by contract* failed to enter public parlance, probably because in the reform era, it was difficult for people to associate contracts—a cherished symbol of law and rationality—with abuse.

As Huang and the EJI's work continued, they found that psychiatry could be abused not only by families but also by public institutions. In some cases, employers allegedly instructed psychiatrists to secretly diagnose "troublemaking" employees and used the diagnoses to demote or hospitalize them.[4] In other cases, persons who sought to complain about local government wrongdoings to higher authorities or Beijing were arrested by local police and thrown into psychiatric hospitals, often under the diagnosis of paranoid schizophrenia (Wu 2016). In response to the negative press coverage on this latter group of cases, Dr. Sun Dongdong, a forensic psychiatrist and professor at Peking University, said in an interview: "The public often thinks that only those people who are disheveled, crazy-looking, and violent are mentally ill. In fact, many mentally ill patients look completely normal except for their psychotic symptoms. As for those veteran petitioners [who keep on petitioning no matter what responses they receive], I can reliably say that, if not 100%, then at least 99% of them are mentally ill, with paranoid psychosis." Thus, he suggested that those "veteran petitioners" be hospitalized because paranoid psychosis would drive them to disrupt the social order (Wang 2009).

Sun's remark spurred an outcry. Many people saw him as denigrating the wretched victims of political injustice and their rightful appeals. Meanwhile, although there had only been a handful of reported cases of alleged wrongful hospitalization,[5] Sun's sweeping claim allowed human rights activists to make general statements about the phenomenon and its underlying causes. They scaled up the target of their criticism from paternalism in families to that of the state, which they argued was manifested in governments' attempts to pathologize the individual and police the social. On Sina Weibo (新浪微博), the Chinese counterpart of Twitter, Huang Xuetao warned the country's leaders against letting their paternalistic desires run wild and trying to *guan* (control) everything.[6] Invoking the Confucian idea of "family-state isomorphism," she said: "State paternalism and cultural paternalism [in the family] are isomorphic . . . Paternalism is boundless in China, with the doctor-patient relationship being the hardest-hit area."[7] As she argued, this is because biomedicine provided hegemonic standards through which our interests and well-being can be evaluated: "We are entitled to make choices only when [biomedicine sees our choices as] rational and correct."[8]

"Being Mentally Illed" and the Normal/Pathological Distinction

Although cases of psychiatric abuse were shocking to the public, activists still hoped the issue would become mainstream and therefore directly concern the populace at large, not just the unlucky bunch who suffered its effects. In this way, the entire citizenry would feel like a stakeholder and this would exert pressure on the legislature. The opportunity came in 2010, when a man named Peng Baoquan was forcibly hospitalized by local police after lodging complaints about his company's corruption to higher authorities and then participating in a protest held by other petitioners. In text messages calling for help, he used the term *bei jingshenbing* (*being mentally illed*) to describe his situation. At the time, there was a trend of adding "被/*bei*," a preposition suggesting the passive voice, to words not typically used passively to show a lack of control, especially vis-à-vis oppressive public powers (公权力/*gong quanli*) or power wielded by government institutions (Hou 2010). For example, when a government corruption whistleblower was found dead, the phrase *being suicided* (被自杀/*bei zisha*) emerged to convey disbelief in the police's claim that it had been a suicide (He 2009). When journalists picked up the phrase *being mentally illed* in reporting Peng's and other cases (Anonymous 2010), it became an instant hit, because it revealed a new level of political vulnerability: one could lose both freedom and the capacity of self-representation when labeled mentally ill. Because *bei* implied the subject's passive victimhood and innocence, it also created the impression—and fear—that *anyone* could fall prey to psychiatric abuse.

Seeing the evocative potential of "being mentally illed," Huang Xuetao and colleagues put it to use. They used it to frame cases of wrongful hospitalization to draw public attention. They also argued in a 2010 legal analysis that the psychiatric system had rendered everyone vulnerable to being mentally illed with its hegemonic and illogical standards such as insight, which saw a person's denial of having mental illness as a manifestation of mental illness (Huang, Liu, and Liu 2010). The report was widely circulated in the media, and it became a text that psychiatrists felt obliged to address. Moreover, on Sina Weibo, Huang mentioned "being mentally illed" over three hundred times, portraying it not as a distant potentiality but as an impending reality for everyone. For instance, when the Chinese National Center for Disease Prevention and Control estimated in 2011 that over sixteen million people in China were suffering from SMIs, she contended that Chinese psychiatrists were trying to label everyone with a diagnosis and subject them to hospitalization. Given that we are all on our way to "being mentally illed," Huang said, we should fight for the rights of those already in the psychiatric system; only then can we protect our own rights.[9]

Though useful, the phrase *being mentally illed* carried implications that activists and allies had not intended. Firstly, while it was used to frame various types of wrongful hospitalization, including family-initiated hospitalization like Chen Dan's, the term's association with other *bei*-phrases tended to highlight the authoritarian state and its abuse of psychiatry, leaving critiques of the family to the side. In fact, in Peng Baoquan's case and in several other cases of alleged wrongful hospitalization of petitioners, activists and allies argued that the procedure was illegal partly because the family had not made the decision and had not even been informed (Gong and Chen 2012). Thus, in those arguments, the family figured to be a haven that could protect the individual from the incursion of state power.

Additionally, the phrase was commonly taken to suggest that the victim was *biologically normal* and should not be subjected to psychiatric diagnosis or hospitalization; it was also seen as implying that those who were *truly mentally ill* should be. Huang and colleagues occasionally endorsed this position, such as in the aforementioned 2010 legal analysis. Moreover, in my conversations with them, most people who sought help from EJI saw themselves as normal individuals who had been coerced into receiving psychiatric treatment; they desperately hoped to have their diagnoses removed and reputations restored through lawsuits. Although EJI staff wanted these survivors of psychiatric hospitalization to fight for patient rights such as self-determination, the exercise of legal capacity, and community inclusion, they did not want to be associated with patients or persons with disabilities and could not care less about these groups' rights. As such, the human rights campaign at the time sidelined individuals who identified themselves as mentally ill and in need of care, and it failed to offer care that could serve as an alternative to psychiatric hospitalization or medication.

Meanwhile, the normal/pathological distinction upheld by "being mentally illed" had left the biomedical logic intact and given psychiatrists the authority to determine who was "truly" mentally ill. In wrongful hospitalization lawsuits, hospital representatives typically asked that the plaintiff be sent for rediagnosis, because they believed that mental illness was chronic with an unpredictable remission and relapse cycle and that hospitalization at any point of the illness trajectory would be justified. The plaintiff's lawyer and human rights activists would object to that request, arguing that mental illness, or at least the condition requiring hospitalization, was temporary and that rediagnosis could not reveal the person's mental status at the time of commitment. As the psychiatric view dominated people's imaginations of mental illness, the courts often granted the hospital's requests, miring the case in a prolonged process of psychiatric examination.

Confronted with these difficulties, Huang Xuetao and colleagues gradually distanced themselves from the concept of "being mentally illed." In high-profile discussions with leading psychiatrists and legal scholars, they drew on ideas from the United Nation's *Convention on the Rights of Persons with Disability* (United Nations General Assembly 2007), which the Chinese government had ratified in 2008, to argue that a person's mental capabilities are multifaceted rather than "all-or-none," as the concept of insight or the normal/pathological distinction would have it. For example, the fact that one lacks the ability to control emotions does not mean that one necessarily lacks the ability to give or refuse consent for psychiatric treatment. In this argument, society needs to recognize the capabilities and autonomy of people with mental illness as well as provide them with support to exercise these capabilities, rather than make decisions for them or even confine them. According to the activists, China should adopt the strict hospitalization criterion of dangerousness popular in Western liberal democracies— that is, involuntary hospitalization should only be applied when a person puts oneself or others in danger; even then, an independent mental health tribunal should review and authorize the commitment request (Large et al. 2008). Another practice that the activists suggested China learn from the West was deinstitutionalization—that is, the closure or drastic downsizing of psychiatric hospitals.[10] Thus, as the activists scaled up cases of wrongful hospitalization to systemic abuse of psychiatry, a matter concerning every citizen, they drew a progressive history of global human rights. From this historical perspective, China, as an authoritarian state and a paternalistic culture, had fallen behind and needed to catch up with Western liberal democracies; it could do so by using legal and institutional reforms to protect the right to autonomy.

Asserting the Right to Health and
Reclaiming State Paternalism

The idea of patient autonomy was not new to Chinese psychiatry. In 1987 and 1990, experts from the World Health Organization (WHO) organized two workshops in China to help psychiatrists prepare and formulate the MHL, where they insisted that psychiatric hospitalization should be voluntary to the greatest extent possible. As Dr. Liu Xiehe recalled in my interview, many workshop participants had been suspicious of this idea, emphasizing that involuntary treatment was necessary for patients without insight. The human rights campaign finally produced a widespread call for autonomy that leading psychiatrists and other MHL framers had to heed.[11] In June 2011, the State Council released a draft MHL for public commentary. Unlike existing municipal regulations, the draft no longer mentioned medical protection hospitalization. Instead, it stipulated that hospitalization should be voluntary in principle, except when persons with mental illness could not recognize or control their own behavior and posed the danger of harming themselves or others or disturbing public order (Chen 2023). Activists criticized the public order criterion for potentially legitimating political abuse of psychiatry.[12] In October that year, the National People's Congress (2011) released another draft for commentary. It required medical personnel to diagnose and treat patients only at clinical facilities, effectively banning the hospital "pick-up" services that many family members, such as Chen Dan's parents, had used. It also deleted any mention of public order but added that patients could be committed in any situation in which failure to commit would be inconducive to treatment. Activists criticized the latter for giving psychiatrists too much decision-making power (Yang 2012). After another round of media pressure, it also disappeared from subsequent drafts and in the law that was ultimately passed.

While making these concessions, the psychiatrists involved in drafting the MHL felt the need to defend their professional practice and vision. They did so by reworking the terms already established by activists and offering a different, but no less appealing, historical perspective of China. In media interviews and public discussions, they acknowledged the phenomenon of "being mentally illed" but rescaled the two sides of the normal/pathological divide that it implied: they conceded that there might be a few normal individuals who were wrongfully hospitalized, but they could turn to other legislation, such as the Tort Law, for help. Meanwhile, many more people were truly mentally ill, and they should be the real subjects of concern for the MHL (Wu and Xie 2011).

To back up such scaling, psychiatrists drew on statistics and mathematical calculations. For example, Dr. Tang Hongyu (2010), a leading forensic psychiatrist and MHL framer, pointed out that among the sixteen million people with SMIs in China, about 10 percent had a tendency toward violence and would require involuntary hospitalization in any legal framework; yet in 2008, only 740,000 people had received inpatient psychiatric treatment. Thus, Tang contended that most instances of involuntary hospitalization had been correctly applied. Moreover, in response to activists' call for deinstitutionalization, psychiatrists often invoked globally authoritative data, such as data from the WHO mental health atlas, to show that the number of psychiatric beds per capita in China was just above the average in low and lower-middle income countries. They argued that it had fallen far behind upper-middle income countries—the strata to which China now belonged—as well as high-income countries (World Health Organization 2011a, 2011b).[13] Their point was that rather than having too much institutionalization, China did not have enough, and there was a "treatment gap" that needed to be closed. Of course, there were problems with the way psychiatrists used these numbers: for instance, even if we accepted their definition of violence, the 10 percent was more likely a lifetime violence rate instead of the rate at any given point; the China profile in the WHO atlas, collected by China's MOH, did not include data on long-term hospital stays or community facilities. In any case, such data presentations allowed psychiatrists to not only "outscale" (Blommaert 2007, 6) the number of people "mentally illed" with the number of those who were "truly mentally ill" but also outscale the need to prevent wrongful hospitalization with the need to develop psychiatric hospitals and provide inpatient treatment, voluntarily or otherwise. The latter, psychiatrists argued, was the need to protect individuals' right to health.

In June 2013, at a workshop in Beijing that discussed legal and ethical issues pertaining to mental health, I witnessed how stakeholders debated the meaning of the right to health and its relationship with the right to autonomy. Drawing on the *International Covenant on Economic, Social, and*

Cultural Rights, Huang Xuetao argued that the right to health entails individuals' freedom to control their bodies and consent to health services; that is, one has the right *not* to be healthy. In response, Dr. Sun Dongdong drew on China's Tort Law to define the right to health as maintaining the integrity of life and raising its quality, contending that it was the foundation for realizing other rights. The point was not which law was more authoritative; rather, whereas the activist saw health as a subjective desire and the right to it as hinged on the possession of autonomy, the psychiatrist saw health as an objective standard for everyone, far outreaching autonomy in importance.

From the perspective of leading psychiatrists, the right to autonomy was not just secondary to the realization of the right to health but potentially antagonistic to it, and the "progressive" global history the activists envisioned was, in fact, regressive. In venues like the aforementioned workshop and my interviews with them, psychiatrists and their allies often discussed the ruin brought about by deinstitutionalization in Western countries: for instance, they discussed the life of Joyce Brown, a homeless woman who had defeated New York City's attempt to forcibly hospitalize her but who later "died with her rights on";[14] they recounted their encounters with desperate overseas Chinese families who had to bring their loved ones with mental illness back to the motherland for treatment and who were indignant about the careless American psychiatric system (Jia 2010). Therefore, whereas activists scaled up cases of abuse to a critique of China's authoritarian and paternalistic regime, psychiatrists scaled up anecdotes of neglect to a critique of the Western world, especially the humanitarian tragedies brought on by its idolization of individual autonomy.

To prevent such humanitarian tragedies from happening in China, psychiatrists endorsed "state paternalism" in the MHL, defining it as the "care and love that society exercises for the sick, the vulnerable, and the disabled" even when they refuse, and they saw it manifest in "the restrictive measures imposed to safeguard patients' interests in health," such as involuntary hospitalization and treatment (Xie and Ma 2011a). They further scaled it up from a matter benefiting just people with mental illness, however many there were, to one relevant to everyone, because it would protect them from potential patient violence and from social ills such as high homelessness rates. Indeed, although disturbance of public order could not be included as a criterion of commitment, psychiatrists and other framers highlighted *guan*— reconfigured as *guanli* (management)—in the MHL, stipulating as a general principle the establishment of a comprehensive management system to prevent and treat mental illness, to rehabilitate and monitor patients (National

People's Congress 2012, Article 6). As psychiatrists saw it, this state paternalism was a feature of the Chinese culture vis-à-vis the West and an advantage of the socialist polity vis-à-vis capitalism (Wu and Xie 2011).

Risk and the Legal Pivot Called "Family"

As a socialist legacy, "state paternalism" in Maoist-era mental health care had focused on community care, and it required the active presence of state agents. In contrast, psychiatrists' invocation of state paternalism during the legislative debates was not only centered on hospitalization but, ironically, it also remained vague about the state's role. In my interview, Dr. Liu Xiehe said that the key issue in the legislation, as he and many colleagues had perceived it, was to have the government provide free treatment to impoverished patients. Nevertheless, when he had started drafting the law in the 1980s, "somebody from above" had told him not to mention anything about money or governmental provision. In the 2013 workshop, Dr. Sun Dongdong also attributed the sluggish legislation process to the fact that mental health was more likely to "burn rather than earn" money for the government. Therefore, psychiatrists equivocated on whose role it was to safeguard individuals' right to health, and the official MHL repeatedly uses *should*—a vague and unenforceable word—to stipulate public sector responsibilities. Without the state's financial and institutional support, how could the MHL meet psychiatrists' call for state paternalism—safeguarding the individual's health as they defined it and protecting the public from potential violence—on the one hand and activists' demand for individual autonomy on the other?

One mechanism for achieving this was the concept of risk. While the activists called for limiting involuntary hospitalization to people who posed an immediate and substantial danger to themselves or others, the MHL frames the criterion in a slightly different—but consequential—way: one may be committed if one has already injured oneself/others *or* "is in danger of endangering" oneself/others (National People's Congress 2012, Article 30). Note that the law does not define what *danger of endangering* means; in fact, a psychiatrist-framer told me that it had been intentionally left vague to allow room for interpretation. Because this concept serves to transform the indefinite and uncertain future into assessment of present action, I suggest that it constitutes what sociologists have called "risk" (Dean 1998).[15] While an actual danger highlights an individual's right to autonomy by delimiting it, the vast and unrealized potentiality of risk incorporates many different concerns, including the protection of autonomy; the taming of pathology to promote biomedically-defined health; and the detection, prevention, and management of social disturbance.

If the risk criterion incorporates the right to autonomy of the "normal" individual and the right to health of the "pathological" subject by being the flexible divide between them, then who should be responsible for reading risk and safeguarding the corresponding right? Unable to hold the state financially accountable for mental health services, the MHL limits public sector interventions to allowing work units and the police to take risky individuals suspected of having mental illness to assessment and to allowing the police to commit people with SMIs who pose risks to others. It also does not require independent mental health tribunals to review commitment requests, as demanded by activists. As Dr. Tang Hongyu stated in my interview, there were no financial resources for setting up such tribunals, and they might be usurped by local governments to authorize psychiatric abuse regardless.

Without public sector involvement, responsibility fell back to the family. During the legislative debates, leading psychiatrists brushed aside cases of wrongful hospitalization by families as rare exceptions to the norm. They claimed that "familial affection (亲情/qinqing) is the kindest of all human emotions,"[16] especially in the family-oriented Chinese culture. Against activists' suggestion that family members could be ill-willed, they argued that family members of people with SMIs in China were "bearing the heaviest responsibility and blame" (忍辱负重/renru fuzhong) in the world (e.g., Xie, Tang, and Ma 2011, 724), as they carried burdens of care and faced the stigma of mental illness without complaint. While the last statement shows that the psychiatrists had some structural awareness of families' circumstances, the overall effect of these culturally essentialist remarks was to cast family members as naturally willing and suitable to carry out the work of care and management.

Indeed, the MHL that these psychiatrists drafted not only fails to alleviate families' burdens, but it can exacerbate them by giving family members a laundry list of responsibilities: to help patients get treatment, provide for daily needs, monitor behavior, facilitate rehabilitation, bear liability in case their denial of treatment leads to patients injuring others, and so on (National People's Congress 2012). Without institutional resources to distribute these responsibilities, all that the psychiatrists could do, as Dr. Tang Hongyu said in my interview, was to grant families rights to match their responsibilities. They wrote in a semifinal draft that family members could take people suspected of having mental illness to assessment, whether or not risk was involved, and that they could commit those with SMIs who posed risks to themselves or others. The State Council and the National People's Congress approved this stipulation and went a step further to rescind the redress procedure that the psychiatrists had designed for people committed by their families: as the final drafts and the official MHL stipulate, these individuals may not request a rediagnosis to overturn the decision recommending their commitment—whereas people committed by the police may do so—and they may not request discharge themselves (Chen 2023).

All responsibilities and rights are congealed in the system of guardianship. The MHL defines *guardians* as "people who may become guardians according to the General Principles of the Civil Law" (National People's Congress 2012, Article 83), including spouses, parents, adult children, other close relatives, and other relatives or friends who are willing to take the responsibilities and who are approved by the person's work unit or neighborhood committee. Under the General Principles of the Civil Law, only adults adjudicated by the court to be lacking or limited in legal capacity would be assigned guardians (National People's Congress 1986, Articles 17–18); in contrast, the MHL assumes that every person with mental illness has a guardian. As another manifestation of guardianship's centrality, the MHL mentions the word *guardian* and its synonyms *family* and *(close) relatives* fifty-two times, more frequently than any other agent.

Note that guardians are not supposed to just rescind the individuals' autonomy and discipline them with the biomedical standards of health. The MHL also grants guardians the right to challenge involuntary hospitalization imposed by the police and requires them to get people who are legally allowed to be released out of the hospital. In these occasions, at least, guardians are supposed to help their loved ones achieve freedom. As such, the family has become a pivot in the MHL, in charge of protecting the sovereign individual's liberty and personal integrity, fostering the normality of the biological subject, and mediating the transition between autonomy and managed health.

Mediation of the Family in Mental Health Care

The MHL has presented a seeming contradiction of simultaneously embracing individual autonomy and family guardianship. My analysis has shown that this strange coexistence is a product of how the family had been constructed and paternalism had been scaled over the past century, as well as the delicate dance in which stakeholders strategically invoked these constructs and scales to advance their agendas and respond to each other in the legislative debates. Beyond strategies, how activists and psychiatrists defined and scaled paternalism reflects two major strands of sociopolitical orientations in contemporary China and their respective assumptions, omissions, and potential concatenations with each other.

Similar to many liberals throughout the country, the activists saw the patriarchal family as a starting point of social critique, but the fear of totalitarianism in the post-Mao era and the influence of international human rights discourses quickly redirected their attention to harm inflicted by the state and its institutions (Lord and Stein 2013). Their assumption and emphasis on individual autonomy, also common in the international human rights circle, made it difficult for them to address vulnerability, interdependence, and complex relations (Nussbaum 2006); at times, they might even come to see the family as a pristine private realm protecting individual autonomy. Meanwhile, the concern for vulnerability was picked up by psychiatrists, who reframed it as a moral to achieve objective standards of biological health through institutional and pharmaceutical treatments (Metzl and Kirkland 2010). They redefined the paternalism in imposing such treatments positively as a socialist legacy enabled by the state. Indeed, underlying their valorization of state paternalism was a desire for a wider distribution of responsibilities for helping individuals achieve health. In the face of deficient state support, however, they had to put these responsibilities squarely on the shoulders of families. Ironically, then, the activists' distaste for state intervention provided psychiatrists and allied policymakers with a convenient excuse for such displacement; in other words, the liberal sentiment against the state was used to justify the state's neoliberal withdrawal from health-care provision.

In the end, the activists' and the psychiatrists' views both found their ways into the MHL, because they were both contained in the ambiguous concept of risk and the family was left to mediate the various rights and subjectivities at stake. Underlying this compromise was the activists' difficulty keeping all the complexities in family care practices firmly in sight. This partly explained the waning of their campaign now that the MHL had supposedly rendered public abuse of psychiatry impossible. It was also the psychiatrists' assumption that family caregivers would always embrace the morals of biomedicine to use institutionalization and medication in alleviating their loved ones' vulnerability. The next few chapters will explore whether, how, and to what extent this is the case.

2

HOSPITALIZATION, RISKS, AND FAMILIAL COMMITMENTS

During my fieldwork, I paid countless visits to the adult psychiatry wards at Benevolence Hospital in the city of Nanhua. Each ward had about ninety patients, the majority of whom had been diagnosed with schizophrenia and the rest with other illnesses such as bipolar disorder or severe depression. The wards were all locked and barred. At night, most patients slept in crowded rooms with ten beds each. A few others lived in double or triple rooms for extra fees, and the rest were put in monitored rooms with their hands or feet tied, either because they were new to the ward and required close observation or because their behavior had been deemed disruptive. In their waking hours, patients—except for the restrained ones—were asked to stay in the large activity room at the center of the ward, under the direct gaze of the nurses' station outside. Each ward had one director, typically four resident psychiatrists, ten or so nurses (working in shifts), and several care workers. Except for the care workers, all the staff had piles of paperwork to do, and they had little time to spend on the ward other than making morning rounds, dispensing medication, or supervising the distribution of meals. Most patients spent their days chatting with each other, watching whatever channel was showing on the TV, or pacing back and forth, talking to themselves. A few of them paid extra fees to go outside the ward for entertainment activities (e.g., gardening and singing). On weekday afternoons or weekends, patients could receive visitors. While city life was roaring right outside the hospital, life on the ward was isolated and dull, but in order.

One patient I met in the hospital was Rong. A thirty-year-old woman, she had converted to Buddhism shortly after her first hospitalization two years before. Back then, her difficult relationship with her boyfriend had made her irritable. She saw ghost-like shadows flying in her room, heard voices talking about her, and felt so scared that she could not help screaming. Thus, she had checked herself into another psychiatric hospital in Nanhua. To her dismay, the pills that the doctors prescribed did not chase away the ghosts but only disturbed her menstrual cycle, which was considered by traditional Chinese medical theories to be an important sign of natural femininity and bodily regeneration.[1] Therefore, she stopped taking the pills after being discharged. One day, she saw the Buddha flying in front of her, telling her how to deal with the ghosts and handle daily tasks. After that experience, she became a Buddhist and had been learning to control her temper through reciting scriptures.

A migrant in the city, Rong had long been living with and supported by her elder sister. Despite her confidence in her own healing practices, Rong's pharmaceutical noncompliance and occasional irritability made her sister worry that she might be relapsing. Her sister suggested that she see a doctor, but she refused. With the excuse of driving her to a family dinner, her sister took her to Benevolence. Weeks into her second hospitalization, Rong was still upset about this arrangement. She complained to me: "I asked her [my sister] to give me a chance, to allow me two or three months without taking pills or being hospitalized [to see if I could control my temper with Buddhist discipline]. Every time I made this request, she refused by saying: 'What if you end up like last time?' I feel like I am just a puppet on a string, being pulled here and there by others. I am not able to resist in the least bit."

Hope, Fear, and Risk: Hospitalization as Intimate Commitment

Rong might be one of the few openly practicing Buddhists on the ward, but she was certainly not alone in having her life derailed by waves of hospitalization and feeling controlled by others. Meanwhile, like Rong's sister, many family members felt that the patient's—or even the whole household's—future was fraught with risks because of mental illness. These risks, they insisted, required constant management through pharmaceuticals and, at times, hospitalization.

In his classical study of the psychiatric asylum, Erving Goffman (1961) urged us to heed inmates' "moral career"—that is, how institutional arrangement and one's position in it constitute one's sense of self. Following his suggestion, I explore how the hospitalization process shapes the patient's illness history, course of treatment, and prognosis, as well as how the self is understood and how people believe it is supposed to develop. Meanwhile, entangled in the hospitalization process are not just patients themselves but also a set of kin relations. As Lawrence Cohen (2013) argued in his study of organ transplants in India, commitment, or giving over a body to another, happens in a particular social relation and moral world "in a way that remakes both its being and its horizon" (319). Taking a cue from Cohen, I explore the vision of life to which family members are committed when committing their loved ones to the hospital; the financial resources, emotional energies, and physical labor they commit; and how inpatient treatment in turn transforms their desire, responsibility, and authority in relation to their loved ones. I focus on hospitalization practices before the passage of the MHL and pay special attention to how they shape families' understandings of risk, an idea that would become central in the law and its implementation.

Rong's story resembles Tingting's, which I described at the beginning of the book. To recap, Tingting was a first-time inpatient who had been disturbed and rendered sleepless by chaotic experiences, both at work and in her love life. Her mother, Mrs. Dong, had put her in the hospital and later decided to pull her out of her job as an attempt to protect her from potential harm and ensure her medication compliance. Both Rong and Tingting were frustrated about their families' interventions. Yet while Mrs. Dong was still trying various intervention measures, Rong's sister, who had been exposed to the psychiatric discourse longer, was committed to one measure—risk management through repeated hospitalizations. This chapter treats the cases of Tingting, Rong, and other inpatients as situated at different points on a common path of intimate involvement in mental health care. I will trace how this path is constructed by psychiatric discourse and hospitalization practices, how caregivers' everyday practices and senses of commitment change along the way, and how families' new biomedical commitments turn them into quasi-psychiatric institutions on the one hand while helping to sustain the psychiatric hospital on the other, reinforcing the hospital-family circuit of mental health care.

Running through this path are uses of the word *guan* when discussing actions toward people with mental illness. As mentioned, *guan* has an underlying cultural meaning as an ethical practice of parenting: parents who *guan* combine discipline and care to protect and train their vulnerable children in the hope that they become fully human, acting in harmony with the social order (Chao 1994) and eventually no longer needing *guan*. For example, while Tingting saw herself as an adult entitled to freedom and no longer bound by *guan*, Mrs. Dong saw Tingting's lifeworld as shattered by madness, turning her into a vulnerable child in need of *guan*. This chapter will examine how desires for *guan*—for developing humans and building order—lead people to the psychiatric hospital in the first place and how the psychiatric reconfiguration of *guan* changes people's hopes and life horizons, generating practical and ethical tension.

Madness, *Guan*, and Quests for Order

During fieldwork, I heard people from all walks of life discuss madness with the word 乱/*luan*, which means messy, chaotic, and disordered. Madness, then, is the disturbance of, and deviation from, the orderly world. In the cases I encountered, some of the eruptions were volcanic and palpable to everyone present, such as a man frantically smashing items at home or even stabbing his parents with a knife. Other disruptions were quieter, such as an adolescent feeling estranged from her parents and drawn to the online world. Sometimes, the disorderly experience emerged as one grappling with a disorderly world full of injurious relations. For instance, Rong's ghostly visions appeared shortly after her boyfriend at the time had abused and threatened her; Tingting could not sleep as she thought about whether, as a woman with a homely appearance, her affection for a male colleague would be requited. In other cases, the order that madness putatively disrupted had been embraced by some parties involved but contested by others. For example, a sixty-year-old man told me that he liked treating friends to meals and giving them money as gifts. He also planned to invest in the housing market by refinancing the apartment he had bought for his son. He saw himself as making wise investments for social and financial gains, but his son saw him as manically squandering money and jeopardizing the whole family's interests. These diverse experiences with and claims of disorder often reflect changing social expectations, gender and generation gaps, precarious interpersonal ties, and feelings of vulnerability in the reform era (Ng 2009).

When chaos is discerned and unbearable, a quest for order follows. The quest can take many forms, sometimes as efforts of self-discipline and self-improvement, sacred or secular. For instance, Rong had turned to the Buddhist cosmological order, hoping that its teachings would allow her to make peace with the spectral beings and herself. Tingting had tried to cool her head by devoting herself to her work, seeking financial and emotional independence. Family members may not understand or sympathize with these efforts, seeing them instead as childish caprices. Thus, they find it necessary to impose their own plans and visions.

In some other cases, patients and families share a common quest for order. For instance, multiple people I spoke with attributed the chaotic experiences to a disturbance or stagnation of *qi*, the life force that, according to traditional Chinese medical theory, generates and regulates all cosmological and bodily functions (Zhang 2007). They associated the patient's behavioral and emotional disturbance with physiological chaos, such as the excessive heat of *fire* (上火/*shanghuo*) in the patient's body. Family members would then use certain foods or herbal concoctions to return the patient's *qi* and its manifestations to a more natural harmony (Ma 2012).

In still other cases, people trace the source of chaos to a disordered family and seek redress for intimate injuries. Perhaps influenced by the newly popular psychological notion that childhood experience shapes, or even determines, one's lifelong well-being (Kuan 2015), many young adults I met attributed the chaos they had experienced to disorders in their natal families, such as frequent fights between their parents. Their family members might agree with those attributions and attempt to adjust the domestic dynamics accordingly by expressing more loving sentiment toward the patients.

Moreover, some women attributed their chaotic experiences to their suffering from gender injustice, sacrifices in love, or sexual exploitation, similar to the "family vernacular" that historian Yumi Kim (2022) discovered as a significant way for Japanese women to discuss madness.[2] For instance, Mei, a woman in her late twenties, told me that she had been driven crazy by love. Soon after moving from an inland province to coastal Guangdong fresh out of high school in 2001, she started a relationship with Mr. Lam, a divorced and well-to-do civil servant with a teenage son. She moved in with him and performed all the housework. With the excuse of protecting his son, however, he called her a "maid" and had her sleep in a separate room when the son returned home from boarding school on weekends. Although she yearned for the recognition of marriage, he told her that they could only marry when his son went to college. Worse still, he forced her to have three abortions over the years. In 2009, she began hearing voices in which people called her a "whore" and was having visions of babies' heads hanging from trees. "After so many years of suffering, I couldn't bear it, and it suddenly exploded," she said in one of our conversations. Of course, not all women on the ward were in a socially ambiguous position like Mei, but many did attribute the chaos they experienced to the intimate injustice they had suffered. The only solution they saw was to have their partners or in-laws acknowledge past mistakes and treat them with more love and appreciation.[3] Perhaps unsurprisingly, the people they blamed typically brushed aside those claims.

Therefore, although madness commonly entails experiences of chaos and disorder, exactly what is disordered and what order needs to be (re)installed are uncertain. As Annemarie Mol (2002) has pointed out, because bodily reality is not fixed but constantly configured in practice, there is "permanent possibility of alternative reconfigurations" (163). She argues that good care is "persistent tinkering in a world full of complex ambivalence and shifting tensions" (Mol, Moser, and Pols 2010, 14). In the face of madness, most people are natural pragmatists, experimenting with various healing options to evaluate which world order (or an emergent hybrid) is most inhabitable, and they often disregard the epistemic differences between these options. A patient might wear a Taoist amulet to drive out evil spirits while also seeking refuge in a hospital. A caregiver might use herbal concoctions to modulate a patient's bodily cycle while also adjusting her interactional style with the patient. Even psychiatrists would sometimes go beyond prescribing pills to intervene in apparent domestic dysfunctions. Dr. Chen, Mei's doctor, repeatedly told Mei's boyfriend that she needed the "emotional warmth from a normal family." These lived experiments may involve different practices, perspectives, and temporal horizons, but they all reflect aspiration for a hopeful future.

It is with this hope that families—and sometimes patients—turn to the psychiatric hospital. A psychiatrist on the ward told me: "Most patients are sent here because their families feel that they are too chaotic (*luan*) to be managed (*guanli*)." This explanation is often found in patients' medical histories, which are typically narrated by family members and recorded by psychiatrists during the intake interview.[4] Compared to other quests for order and other efforts of *guan*, psychiatry seems to provide a "quick fix." As a mother remarked, "We [my husband and I] thought she [our daughter] would be okay after a simple physical exam and taking a few pills."

In fact, the psychiatric industry encourages, and even incites, this hopeful investment in biomedicine. For example, figure 2.1 is an advertisement

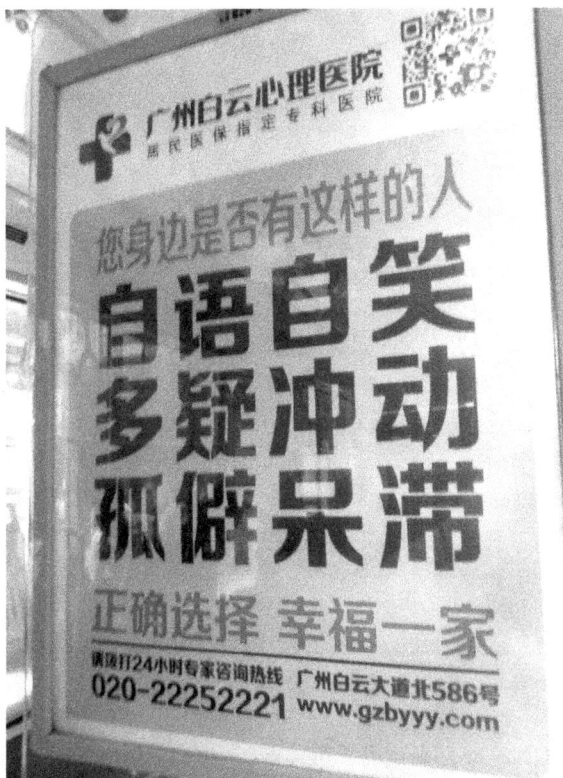

FIGURE 2.1. Bus poster advertisement for a psychiatric hospital. Photo by Zhiying Ma.

posted on a bus, headlined by the name of a psychiatric hospital. It asks: "Is there such a person around you? They talk and laugh to themselves; they are suspicious and impulsive; they are aloof and dull." As you start thinking of such a person in your life and wondering what to do, the ad tells you to "make the right choice, make the family happy," which you can presumably achieve by turning to psychiatry. By urging people to "make the right choice," the ad suggests a contrast between psychiatry and other ways of dealing with the disorder. It implies that psychiatry can determine the nature of the disorder, leaving no place for uncertainty and multiplicity. Moreover, while people often tinker with family dynamics to build a more orderly world for the patient, the ad offers an opposing claim, suggesting that treating one person can secure happiness for the entire family. How does psychiatry justify this claim, and how does it deliver on this promise? What order does it seek to build, and what horizon of life and relations does it open?

To build a dominant order of life-worlds, psychiatrists first need to translate signs of chaos into symptoms of mental illness. They typically take the signs that family members provide as clues to discover more symptomatic behavior, thoughts, or feelings. For example, after learning about Tingting's sleeplessness and mood swings from her mother, Dr. Liu asked Tingting what had kept her up at night and disturbed her. Tingting said it was the thought that her colleagues had all been gossiping about her appearance, laughing at her attempt to pursue love, and conspiring to embarrass her. Dr. Liu told her mother that there was no way everybody could be so focused on her, so he diagnosed her with paranoid schizophrenia. Here, and in many other cases, psychiatrists act as guards of reality, against which they judge patients' thoughts and perceptions.

In their search for patients' mental distortions, psychiatrists perceive many barriers: patients may lack knowledge of their own mental processes; they may be unable to describe it; or worse still, they may deliberately hide it to evade treatment. Therefore, psychiatrists often feel the need to play linguistic games of suggestion, elicitation, and confrontation with patients. For instance, Yun, a thirty-year-old woman who had previously been hospitalized for schizophrenia, had recently been readmitted by her mother-in-law. The latter found it strange that whenever others suggested Yun visit her natal home, she would protest and burst out crying. On the ward, the doctor asked Yun why this was the case. Sobbing, she responded: "I'm not sick. I just don't want to see my father. He used to drag me to the [psychiatric] hospital, so I am really scared of him. Also, he has cheated on my mother and treated her badly." Unable to elicit Yun's cooperation in producing a mental, rather than familial, disorder, the doctor drew in other signs provided by Yun's in-laws and her previous medical records, especially the fact that she had been troubled by visions of ghosts before. The doctor suggested, "You didn't want to go visit your father's home because you saw dirty [i.e., unearthly] things there, right?" Yun denied this assertion, claiming that she had always hated her father. The doctor then confronted her in an angry tone: "Well, that's not true. You lived with your parents for quite a while after you got married, and you even worked for your father by collecting rents for his properties. It was only when you got sick that you avoided him!"

The doctor might have seen herself as a detective trying to catch the patient in a lie. If we follow Mol's idea and view reality as open to multiple configurations, however, then Yun's case illustrates different parties' divergent efforts to configure the reality of dis/order: while the patient spoke in a family vernacular and attributed the disturbing signs (e.g., her emotional refusal to visit her natal home) to a disorder of kin relations, the psychiatrist translated the signs into a mental disorder, which putatively prevented Yun from being a filial daughter. Psychiatric translations like this reduce possible readings of the disorder to a single interpretation and locate it firmly in the patient's mind. Their strategies echo the promise in the ad: only when the individual is treated by psychiatry can order and happiness be restored to the entire household.

After translating the disturbing signs into symptoms of a mental disorder, psychiatrists further reduce it into a neurochemical disorder. Contemporary Chinese psychiatry, like its international counterparts, is dominated by the receptor theory. This theory attributes mental disorders to malfunctioning neurotransmitter pathways and to altered levels of dopamine, serotonin, or glutamate in the brain. Treatment entails manipulating the corresponding neurochemical receptors with drugs such as clozapine, perphenazine, and risperidone (Maddux and Winstead 2019). Most psychiatrists I interviewed devoutly follow this theory, and they see the neurochemical malfunctions as determined by genetic factors. They might recognize the role of dysfunctional domestic lives, gender injustice, or other psychosocial processes in triggering disorders, but they tend to regard these factors only as stressors that induce expressions of the underlying genetic predispositions. Compared to genetics and neurotransmitters, these psychosocial stressors appear to be less specific, generalizable, researchable, and real.[5] This perspective was captured in a psychiatrist's response when I asked what kinds of stress would cause mental disorders: "Many people say the onset is due to great pressure or stressors, but how can there be so many stressors? These are not the key problems. The key is biological."

Under this view, a psychiatrist's job is to use psychopharmaceuticals to reorder patients' neurochemical levels and control their symptoms. The psychiatrist still needs to do a lot of tinkering, but mostly with drug types and dosages (sometimes together with other neurological treatments such as modified electroconvulsive therapy), and the goals are to modulate patients' symptoms and to confirm or overturn a tentative diagnosis. For example, for a patient who is both suicidal and hallucinating, the fact that antidepressants, rather than antipsychotics, work to keep both symptoms at bay suggests a diagnosis of severe depression with secondary psychosis rather than schizophrenia. Moreover, psychopharmaceuticals, especially antipsychotics, usually carry with them various side effects, such as obesity, diabetes, extrapyramidal reactions (i.e., repetitive, involuntary movements), and endocrine dyscrasia (e.g., irregular menstruation). Tinkering with drugs can hopefully help psychiatrists maximize the effects of symptom control and minimize the side effects, ensuring treatment safety and medication compliance.

Aside from prescribing drugs, psychiatrists also use conversation to inculcate insight in patients so that they can distinguish symptomatic thoughts and emotions from the biomedically defined reality and recognize their need for treatment. One day during ward rounds, Dr. Chen told Rong, "I'm not against you practicing Buddhism, but you should know that the voices of gods and ghosts are caused by mental illness." Then she pointed to a disheveled woman across the activity room who kept murmuring to a ghost, laughing, and crying to herself. "Normal people aren't like that," Dr. Chen said. "If you don't want to end up like her, work with me. Let me know what you see and how you feel, but don't stop taking your meds." Rong pushed back by saying that the meds made her stop having periods, which in turn made her irritable. Dr. Chen promised to adjust the dosage and use other drugs to alleviate the side effects, but she insisted that irregular menstruation was merely a *side* effect, not a pathogenic factor. "The main thing right now is to control your symptoms," she emphasized. "The periods will come back once you're cured and stop taking the medications. Anyway, isn't it better not to have periods?" Like Dr. Chen, most psychiatrists welcome, or even solicit, patients' reports of side effects. Yet as they see it, an insightful patient should trust that psychiatrists can manage these side effects; if not, they are the necessary price to pay for reestablishing mental order.

This psychiatric ordering of the patient's life is facilitated by the ward's spatial and social order. As I observed at Benevolence, patients' schedules were carefully regimented. Four times a day, they would line up in front of a nurse in the activity room. One by one, they received a small box of pills, swallowed them on the spot, and opened their mouths so that the nurse could check for hidden pills. In their spare time, psychiatrists encouraged them to chat and interact with each other, lest they withdraw into their disorderly minds. Yet except for receiving friends and family members who came to visit, patients were forbidden from contacting the outside world, which psychiatrists saw as a source of disturbance to the ordering efforts inside. In this sterile environment, it was considered ideal if patients could develop insight and willingly comply with the treatment. If they dared to challenge the order of the ward or if their symptoms became too disruptive to be controlled by pharmaceuticals, then the staff would resort to restraint, such as putting them in the monitored room and tying them to the bed.

Understandably, most patients consider the occasional restraints and everyday regimentations to be a form of control, and they protest their subjugation. As psychiatrists see it, these measures reflect a benevolent *guan*: like parents caring for children, they commit themselves to promoting patients' well-being by striving to bring order back to patients' lives. Given their professional expertise, *guan* in the hospital may be preferable to *guan* at home, especially if home life has been rendered precarious. For example, when a patient—a migrant worker living alone in the city—begged his doctor to discharge him, the doctor tried to comfort him by saying: "Here there are people looking after (*guan*) you, and there are routines in your life, whereas at home everything is messed up. [So just stay here,] okay?"

As such, hospitalization redefines *guan* and, at least temporarily, transfers its authority away from the family. In countries like India (Pinto 2014), Japan (Kim 2022), and Mexico (Reyes-Foster 2018), family members are allowed, or even required, to stay with patients in the psychiatric hospital to provide care. In contrast, once family members in China authorize patients' commitment and provide illness narratives for doctors to make a diagnosis, they do not, or are not supposed to, have much influence on inpatient treatment. At Benevolence, the staff would sometimes ask family members to come to the ward and learn about patients' progress, provide consent for certain treatment, or pay unpaid bills. Yet the staff did not like frequent family visits, lest their pluralist and often nonbiomedical quests for order jeopardize the psychiatric ordering of patients' lives. The staff was also concerned that, with their emotional ties to patients, family members might yield to patients' supplications for discharge too easily: they might perceive the treatment measures as cruel and fail to see the benefits; or, overjoyed by temporary symptom improvements, they might rush to return patients home without realizing that it takes time for the biomedical order to set in. For example, Mrs. Dong saw Tingting's disorder as partly associated with a nutritional imbalance that had made her obese, self-conscious, and emotionally unstable. On the ward, Mrs. Dong brought Tingting home-cooked meals every day, asked if Dr. Liu could add nutritional supplements to her prescriptions, and complained that the antipsychotics were making Tingting even bigger. Annoyed by these requests and complaints, Dr. Liu chastised Mrs. Dong for being too anxious and for intervening (*guan*) too much. From the psychiatric perspective, once family members commit patients to the hospital, they should step back, suspend their emotional attachments or alternative epistemologies, and let biomedicine—the only right measure of *guan*—work its magic.

Anticipating Hope, Apprehending Risks

Although the ad in figure 2.1 promises a simple cure, recovery turns out to be more complex. While many family members bring their loved ones to the hospital in search of a "quick fix," to psychiatrists, recovery entails a protracted process and a different meaning. At Benevolence, psychiatrists would routinely inform patients and family members of three phases in treating schizophrenia and other SMIS: acute, stabilization, and maintenance. The acute phase is the first six to eight weeks after symptom onset, during which immediate inpatient treatment and a high dose of drugs should be used to alleviate the symptoms. The next four to six months are the stabilization phase, during which a moderate dose of drugs should be used to solidify the treatment effects, and the patient can be gradually transitioned back home. The final phase is for maintenance, during which symptoms may be less severe or even absent, but a lower dose of drugs should be continued to prevent relapse. For patients with only one episode, the maintenance phase is one to two years; the more relapses they have, the longer this phase has to last.

By depicting an increasingly obstinate disorder, this advice reflects the idea of degeneration that has been central to the notion of schizophrenia for over a century, since the German psychiatrist Emil Kraeplin developed the concept of dementia praecox (Shorter 1998). More recently, neurobiological studies in global psychiatry have traced patients' cognitive and behavioral degeneration through the toxic brain states that episodes of mental disorder produce (Andreasen et al. 2011). In a family education workshop, the chair of Benevolence's adult psychiatry department drew on these studies and showed the audience a series of MRI scans of the brain of a patient with schizophrenia at different points of his illness trajectory. Pointing to the pictures, he said: "Look, the more relapses the patient has, the more his brain shrinks."[6] The withered organ at the end of the timeline looked grisly, and he framed it as the worst-case scenario, not as the definite future of every patient. In addition, psychiatrists at Benevolence typically gave family members the following prognosis: among all patients with schizophrenia, a third will completely recover with no relapse or need for more medication. Another third will experience a clinical cure and partial recovery; that is, their major symptoms will subside, and with only minor symptoms or small-scale relapses, they can manage their everyday lives with medication. The final third of patients, however, will face frequent relapses and complete degeneration.

We can see that while people commonly perceive madness to be a palpable and temporary disorder in and of the present, the psychiatric discourse puts mental illness on a chronic trajectory. Even after symptoms have disappeared, the degeneration narrative and the longitudinal brain scans remind us that the disorder persists, that the brain damage is irreversible (although in mild cases it may be negligible), and that the patient's condition may deteriorate insidiously. The statistical prognosis then turns this uncertain future of mental disorder into a calculable estimate of probability. The difference between hopeful recovery and fearful degeneration becomes a function of the number, duration, and severity of relapses, which in turn are influenced by an array of risk factors. In this way, the prognosis diverts our attention from the presence (or absence) of symptoms to a "future as that which matters" (Adams, Murphy, and Clarke 2009, 249). This produces "a knowledge that the truth about the future can be known by way of the speculative forecast, itself relying on proliferating modes of prediction" (247).

The future of chronicity and probable degeneration requires present action. As Sarah Lochlann Jain (2007) points out, while prognosis provides a stunningly specific prediction at the patient population level, it is bloodlessly vague when it comes to the individual. In the case of SMIs, one does not know—and may never know until the patient's death—to which third the patient belongs. Thus, the Janus-faced prognosis encourages efforts to move the patient from one category of fate to another. At Benevolence, psychiatrists regularly told family members that they had to continue monitoring patients' risk factors—medication noncompliance, sleep problems, mood swings, and so on—throughout the maintenance phase and for the rest of patients' lives. If present, they should promptly bring these risks under control, preferably through rehospitalization, or else the patients would relapse and degenerate even further.

Such admonition of risk monitoring entangles people's hope with fear. To pursue a better biomedical future for the patient, one must constantly watch for and eliminate signs of risk. This vigilance of risk, as Vincanne Adams and colleagues (2009) stated, is a strategy to avoid "surprise, uncertainty and unpreparedness, but it is also a strategy that must continually keep uncertainty"—including the fear and anxiety that it produces—"on the table" (250). To escalate this vigilance, in recent years, psychiatrists around the world have been promoting the idea of early detection. This involves identifying high risk factors (e.g., family history of mental illness), reducing precipitating factors (especially the psychological stress induced by negative emotional expressions from parents), and recognizing prodromal symptoms before an acute outbreak (e.g., erratic behavior or an aloof personality; Maddux and Winstead 2019). This idea of early detection has influenced psychoeducation materials and advertisements such as that in figure 2.1, which highlight personality traits and behavioral characteristics that are perhaps unwelcome but certainly not uncommon and that few would readily identify as madness. This has expanded the range of risks that have to be monitored. Similarly, psychiatrists at Benevolence would routinely ask family members during intake interviews if patients had displayed such strange behavior or personality traits before the onset of symptoms, even in their early childhoods, and if they had relatives with mental illness or who were "just a little off." These practices of recall did not so much influence the current treatment as help to construct a history of bad genes and missed signs. This history then generated feelings of desperation and urgency among family members: even if patients had been hospitalized following symptom outbreak, the disease might have been secretly progressing for years. Therefore, family members should spare no effort in preventing the situation from deteriorating, and they should make sure not to miss any signs of risk in the future.

Risk Management and Intimate Commitments

Now that the psychiatric "quick fix" has become a chronic task of risk management, how is this task implemented in interactions within and beyond the walls of the psychiatric hospital? Although psychiatrists repeatedly ask them to stick to their meds, many patients I have encountered stop complying soon after they leave the hospital: they either do not think of themselves as suffering from mental illness, or they cannot bear the medications' heavy side effects. After all, the side effects, such as drooling, shaky hands, menstrual irregularity, and drowsiness, might not only make the person feel miserable but also become visible signs of mental illness, incurring stigma and even social exclusion on the person. Because of patients' refusal of the pharmaceutical regimens, family members often must make return visits to the hospital on their behalf, report their emotional, physical, or behavioral changes to the doctors, and receive updated prescriptions. To ensure their everyday medication compliance and to keep an eye on them, some families would ask patients to quit their job or school and stay at home, and a family member would also need to stay at home with them. This person is usually a retired parent or a female relative, especially one who works in a low-income, flexible occupation and whose job is seen as dispensable or secondary to her "natural" task of caregiving. For example, upon receiving the doctor's advice on continued risk management, Mrs. Dong decided to both quit her own job as a restaurant manager and resign on Tingting's behalf. She proposed to open an herbal tea stall with Tingting to look after her.

Understandably, families' decisions to rearrange patients' lives and to keep them at home may frustrate patients, making them feel suffocated and infantilized. Such practices do not delight the "controlling" party either. The hospital bills and income changes may plunge the family into poverty. The primary caregiver may become economically dependent on other family members and vulnerable to their blame if anything goes wrong with the patient. Moreover, unlike the hospital staff, many caregivers are either unable or unwilling to use force on patients, so the question of "How should I *guan*?" preoccupies them every day. For instance, to get the patients to take their meds, caregivers often engage in trivial, yet painful, negotiations with them. They either dole out "bribes" such as soft drinks, cigarettes, and money, or mix ground pills with patients' meals while fearing discovery. To prove that the pills are not poisonous, they sometimes even have to take the pills themselves in front of the patients.

We can see that the psychiatric task of risk management divides the family into the managed and the manager. The managing agents must commit constant emotional energy, physical labor, and financial resources to ensuring medical compliance of the managed and keeping mental illness at bay. When caregivers interrupt patients' life trajectories and keep them at home under watch, families in effect become totalizing institutions that enclose and control patients. Yet this task of risk management also subjects caregivers to economic precarity, homebound lives, and misunderstanding or hostility from patients and other family members.

How, then, do families' newfound commitments to risk management sustain the psychiatric institution? In his analysis of the American pharmaceutical industry, Joseph Dumit (2012) argued that the traditional concept of health as an absence of illness has been replaced by a new concept of health as risk reduction. Operating under this new concept, the "expert patients" constantly watch for their risks of future illnesses and use pharmaceuticals to modulate these risks. Ironically, this practice of risk reduction proliferates the risks that one discovers, thereby helping to maximize pharmaceutical prescriptions and Big Pharma's profits. Similarly, Mary-Jo DelVecchio Good (2001) has suggested that the "biotechnical embrace" of patients enables financial flows to medicine. In our case, it is the caregiver rather than the patient who is trained to embrace biomedicine and its risk logic, but caregivers' biomedical commitments likewise contribute to, and are in turn shaped by, psychiatric profits.

In many of the hospitals I visited, doctors and nurses spent much time calculating how many inpatients they had and how much money they were making on each patient. This is because hospitals—including those funded by the government—all require and count on their clinical units to generate profits, and the revenue each unit produces directly influences its staff's income, especially bonuses. While many doctors see both inpatients and outpatients, inpatients are far more profitable than outpatients. Partly because of this, many doctors tend to recommend hospitalization to family members, even when the latter consider the situation to be manageable at home. In April 2014, six months after Tingting's discharge, I accompanied Mrs. Dong on a return visit to Benevolence. It turned out that she was unable to get Tingting involved in running the herbal tea stall. Without a job, Tingting had been staying in her room all day, playing video games and watching pornography online. That day at the outpatient clinic, Mrs. Dong explained Tingting's condition to Dr. Liu and eagerly inquired what kind of adjustment would be needed for her daughter to get better. The response she got was simple: "It looks like your daughter's illness has aggravated. Why don't you just send her here [as an inpatient]?"

When I left the field three months later, Mrs. Dong had yet to send her daughter back to the hospital. Nevertheless, psychiatrists' advice does lead some families to gradually lower their thresholds for risk perception and hospitalization. For example, both Rong and Yun agreed that their initial admissions had been justified, because at that time they had been haunted by ghostly visions. What they resented was that over time, their family members had come to interpret even the little things they did—such as Rong's occasional irritation and pharmaceutical noncompliance or Yun's sleeplessness and "personality change" (i.e., unwillingness to visit her father)—as indicative of risk of relapse, and therefore decide to rehospitalize them. Sometimes, even psychiatrists view certain family members as overreacting. Dr. Chen once said this about the father of a forty-year-old woman: "Oh boy, whatever she does, he will say she's sick. This time, just because she soaked a dirty pillow in water, he said she was relapsing and sent her back here!" What Dr. Chen did not realize was that the father's intolerance of, and overreaction to, his daughter's odd behavior had been conditioned by the psychiatric logic of risk management. As the father told me in an interview, for many years, he had been a regular participant in the hospital's family education workshops and an avid reader of popular guidebooks on psychopathology; these teachings had formed the basis of his decisions.

In any case, no matter how unnecessary psychiatrists perceive a family-initiated commitment to be, they typically consider it morally and technically justified, because it is better to be safe than sorry. Teresa Kuan (2015) argued that contemporary Chinese parenting is an "art of disposition"—that is, "a moral practice that simultaneously recognizes the embedment of human activity while locating opportunities for strategic manipulation" (21). It requires parents to detect, intervene in, and create conditions for child development in a timely manner. This emphasis on timely action is also apparent in family members' decisions to hospitalize patients and in psychiatrists' support for such decisions, except that in our case, the "art of disposition" is shaped by the psychiatric temporality, which considers it never too soon to act.

To secure timely hospitalization for the often-unwilling patient, some family members resort to brute force. During fieldwork, I witnessed several cases in which family members literally dragged a struggling individual to the hospital, but many families do not view this as a viable option. They want to maintain good family relations and have their loved ones perceive their *guan* as benign. After all, individuals who are forcefully committed may not trust their family members anymore. In a few cases, the individuals even threatened to kill their family members if the latter dared to send them to the hospital again. To avoid such rancor, some family members opt for deception. For example, they may tell patients that they are going to the hospital for a brief check-up, and then attribute the hospitalization decision to the doctor, as we saw in Tingting's case. If neither deception nor force by families works, the hospital is ready to help. Before the passage of the Mental Health Law, many psychiatric hospitals in China routinely offered "pick-up services" to families. As we saw in Chen Dan's case, family members could pay to have hospital employees—often equipped with a vehicle, ropes, and sedatives—come to their home (or any preferred place) and transport the person they saw as mentally ill directly to the hospital ward. During the process, the family members could either help or stand aside, pretending to be uninvolved. These "pick-up services" connected the hospital and the family into a closed circuit, allowing it to operate with no hiccups.

No matter how the patient is committed, and no matter how smoothly the hospital-family circuit runs, many family members would readily admit that the hospitalization process is cruel to the patient. They feel that they must harden their hearts and do it, just like parents must harden their hearts to *guan* their young children. They initiate or carry out the commitment, hoping that this time the patient would finally be stabilized, if not cured, and that the patient could be moved from one prognostic category to another, no matter how dim the hope is.

Paths Converging, Paths Diverging

As suggested by their similar frustration, Rong and Tingting were walking— or rather, being taken—along a similar path constructed by the psychiatric discourse and hospitalization practices. After briefly trying out psychiatric treatment, Rong resisted it and turned to Buddhism for a more viable avenue to order; meanwhile, her sister, who had accompanied her to the hospital, became attached to the idea of biomedical risk management, regarding it as the only legitimate form of care. In Tingting's case, hospitalization was just one of her mother's many attempts to bring her life back to order. Yet as they interacted with the hospital and its staff, the biomedical future, in which the patient would be closely and continuously managed by kin, was slowly becoming the only horizon for Tingting and her family.

In the language of *guan*, we can describe this path as follows: drawing on the cultural ideology of parenting, family members (and sometimes patients) initiate an aspirational journey seeking to transform chaos into order, a vulnerable being into a fully functional human. Practices of *guan* take many forms, among which is psychiatry. Psychiatry promises a quick fix that cures the patient and brings happiness to the family by translating diverse experiences of madness into symptoms of an ontological mental disorder, treating it with drugs and institutional discipline. At the same time, psychiatry also teaches people to see risks in everyday life and to anticipate a fearful future of degeneration. This entanglement of hope and fear reconfigures family members' pluralistic attempts of *guan* into perpetual risk management, which entails medication oversight, repeated hospitalizations, and the rearrangement of lives for patients—and themselves. In this way, the family becomes a quasi-psychiatric institution, and its practices also help sustain the discourse and institution of psychiatry.

Of course, psychiatry cannot exhaust reality as it claims to. On the ward, patients and families are already questioning, resisting, or tinkering with the psychiatric diagnoses and treatment. Outside the hospital, psychiatry's grasp may be even less complete, as people need to find ways to be with each other and address the multiple forms of vulnerability they face, including the permeation of risk and the potential loss of hope partly conditioned by biomedicine.

3

KINSHIP AND ITS LIMITS AMID
SERIOUS MENTAL ILLNESS

Now that psychiatry has highlighted patients' chronic risk and caregivers' chronic responsibility, let us examine how they shape the making and breaking of family ties. In India, Veena Das and Renu Addlakha (2001) have discovered that people may either "seek to localize and isolate disability within the body of one person" or situate disability "within networks of connected kin." They argue that by granting or denying kin membership, these practices help to construct different forms of "domestic citizenship," or intimate belonging with public import (527). In addition, Sarah Pinto (2014) finds that psychiatric care often mediates the dissolution of marriage for women, "add[ing] vulnerability to the already—and inherently—vulnerable condition of kinship" (30). In China, market reform and ideological transformations since the 1980s have brought significant changes to family ties, such as the continued shrinkage of family size, the rising appeal of conjugal intimacy, the prevalence of only children, the obsession with childrearing, the naturalization of care as women's responsibility, and relatedly, the exacerbation of male domination. Inspired by scholars' insight, the first half of this chapter traces how the hope and fear that psychiatry generates reworks the fragility, resilience, and power dynamics of various family relations. Although the biological risk and debility that psychiatry highlights are supposed to affect people of all genders, I examine how they may intersect with existing gender inequalities and hegemonic gender identities—such as what it means to be a woman—to create differential exclusions and subordination (Connell and Messerschmidt 2005). By examining the kinds of domestic citizenship available to or withheld from people diagnosed with SMIs, the analysis illuminates the preconditions and limits hidden in different family relations.

Despite its important role in shaping family relations, psychiatry is not all there is for households. After all, it may not only fail to offer a cure but may also fall short in addressing people's diverse experiences and needs. In everyday life, the household often becomes what Cheryl Mattingly (2014) calls a "moral laboratory," in which people engage with "an uneasily coexisting 'assemblage' of ideals and practices" to produce "singular acts that transform material and social space and create moral selves" (8). For example, in Japan, Ellen Rubinstein (2018) discovered that while parents of persons with SMIs typically rely on biomedical knowledge to shift blame away from themselves and seek help for their children, they also encourage their children to go beyond patienthood and experience the richness of social relationships, and they learn to adapt to their children's unusual behaviors. These experiments in and through the moral laboratories of families may extend, disrupt, or redefine normalcy as constructed by psychiatry, and they may generate what Rayna Rapp and Faye Ginsburg (2011) have called new "kinship imaginaries"—that is, the ways in which family members live with, and construct meanings of, differences together.

The second half of this chapter will explore the kinds of kinship imaginaries these moral laboratories construct and how family members draw on, reframe, or resist ideas of normalcy to build inhabitable worlds (Friedner and Cohen 2015), with or without patients. This contributes to ongoing discussions in disability studies about how families and other forms of intimacy are implicated in forces of normalization or how they can act to complicate or "crip" them (Kim 2017; Rembis 2017). Because care work is unevenly distributed among family members, concentrated heavily on women, I explore the fault lines in these kinship imaginaries, particularly any gender patterns that emerge. This attention to gendered care work and its varying relations to normalcy can explicate what causes caregivers to embrace or depart from the paternalism that psychiatry expects of them, as well as its costs and limitations.

The Fragility of Conjugality

Scholars have pointed out that in reform-era China, the conjugal tie has trumped the parent-child relationship to become the family's central axis, and romantic attachments have replaced filial obligations to become the foundations of family affects (Yan 1997). Conjugal intimacy is supposed to provide people—ideally, everyone—with unconditional and unending love, thereby constituting a haven from the uncertain and self-interested market. Nevertheless, my fieldwork shows that when faced with the risk and responsibility posed by SMIS, people make all kinds of calculations about actual or potential conjugal ties with patients. Thus, conjugality's mixing with market calculations, especially the exclusionary effects this produces, generates much anxiety and heartbreak (Zelizer 2005).

The exclusionary effects are most strongly felt when the spouse/partner decides to leave the patient. In the previous chapter, I mentioned Mei, a woman who had hallucinations after having undergone three abortions for her boyfriend, Mr. Lam, who still denied her marital recognition. An orphan and a migrant worker in Nanhua, she had relied on Mr. Lam for social and economic support. Yet when she was on the ward, Mr. Lam contemplated sending her back to her hometown, where her next-of-kin were all deceased, as soon as she was discharged. He explained his rationale in my interview: "From articles online, I know that only 30% of patients can completely recover from a disease like hers without further relapse. I'm really gambling right now. If I hedge a bet on the 30% side [i.e., Mei's recovery], we'll live together, but I'll face a lot of risks. After all, human beings follow the pleasure principle."

Here, the biomedical logic works with market rationality to legitimize the withdrawal of love. If, as in market transactions, one enters an intimate relationship to seek personal gain and pleasure, then the psychiatric prognosis allows one to adjust his investment in the relationship based on "routinized likelihoods, hedged bets and probable outcomes" (Adams, Murphy, and Clarke 2009, 247). Because the prognosis for SMIS is generally grim, it is unsurprising when a "rational" person, a homo economicus, is unwilling to risk his own future by living with a patient who might relapse repeatedly or degenerate completely. Note that this legitimation is premised on an assumption: mental illness is the patient's own problem. Yet other people, especially the patient herself, may speak a "family vernacular" (Kim 2022) and attribute her disorder to an unjust relation. Perhaps sensing his cold attitude, Mei told Mr. Lam in anger and tears during one of his visits: "I'm sick like this because you were not kind enough to me. After so many abortions [I have undergone for you], there's a huge shadow in my heart. That's why I was paranoid. Do you understand?" Through these charges, Mei demanded that Mr. Lam recognize her intimate sacrifice and repay his relational debt. What Mr. Lam saw as his free and rational choice, then, would appear to Mei as cruel abandonment.

Of course, psychiatry works in multiple ways, and it may allow practitioners to sympathize with and offer help to the patient. After learning about Mr. Lam's intention to leave Mei, many staffers on the ward were indignant. As a pregnant woman who, like Mei, also came from a poor background, Dr. Chen decided to intervene. During Mr. Lam's visits, she repeatedly reminded him of Mei's need for the warmth and love of a family, the lack of which had contributed to bringing about Mei's illness. Meanwhile, immersed in biomedical reductionism, she could not avoid individualizing the illness and seeing the patient as a burden to others: she not only emphasized to Mei the importance of medication compliance but also advised Mei to return to work after discharge, because a man might fear prolonged dependence. In any case, Dr. Chen's hope for Mei's recovery and her plea for Mr. Lam's intimate responsibility were hard to sustain in the face of the risk and chronicity highlighted by psychiatry, as well as the self-interestedness cultivated by the market economy. One day when Dr. Chen was trying to give Mr. Lam a moral lesson, he brushed it off by saying, "Come on. I'm not a savior!" After he left, a doctor who had overheard the conversation commented: "I don't know why you all are so upset with him. If I were him, I would also abandon Mei!"

This happened in 2009.[1] In 2014, right before leaving the field, I ran into Mei again at Benevolence. I was happy to find that she had finally married Mr. Lam and had given birth to a son. She told me that her father-in-law had been kind to her and had forbidden his son from leaving her because of the sacrifices and suffering she had endured. Mei was still uncertain about her future because she had just been rehospitalized, this time for postpartum depression. During my seven years of fieldwork, no one besides Mr. Lam had so vocally expressed a calculated desire to end their relationship with a patient. As I learned from interviews, quite a few patients' spouses or partners—men and women alike—simply walked away from their relationships quietly.

Even when the relationship is still in place, the person's new identity as a chronically risky subject may conflict with normative gender roles in the home. After all, the household is a key productive and reproductive unit in the reform era. Women, in particular, are expected to maintain its everyday operations through childbirth and housework, as the biological and cultural discourses have coalesced to emphasize their "natural" duties as wives and mothers (Evans 1996; Song 2012). Recall Yun, the woman who was hospitalized for refusing to visit her natal home. She told me that she had done this to endear herself to her husband's family. Eight years prior, after her first psychotic episode, her in-laws, who had been living with her, had sent her back to her natal home so that her parents could look after her. Yet her father kept sending her to the hospital, and she found the lengthy separation from her husband unbearable. She was especially worried that her lack of children would make her fall from grace with her husband's family, for she had overheard her mother-in-law suggesting to her husband that he divorce her and find a new wife. To prove her worthiness, she moved back to her marital home, stopped taking the antipsychotics that might complicate pregnancy, and did housework day and night. To her dismay, her mother-in-law saw all of these efforts as signs of an impending relapse—indicating medication incompliance, sleeplessness, delusion, and possible mania—and they only earned her another hospitalization. Together, her patienthood and her marital duties had entrapped her in an impenetrable predicament.

In the psychiatric discourse and its popular readings, a female patient is at risk of not only relapse but also emotional instability, deterioration of mental capacity, and passing down "bad genes" to her children. As my fieldwork shows, pregnant women who are diagnosed with SMIs might be forced into abortion by their husbands' families because of the latter's concern with heredity. Women who already have children might be excluded from everyday childrearing tasks within marriage or denied child visitation after divorce, because they are seen as unfit for mothering. Moreover, women who desire to marry often struggle with whether to disclose their diagnoses to their partners, because disclosure may lead to an immediate breakup, while concealment may generate continued anxiety of being discovered and "dumped." Their doctors' and relatives' advice varies: some tell them not to date at all to avoid heartbreak, while others encourage them to grasp the relationship opportunity first and conceal the diagnosis as long as possible. These responses may come from a sense of protection, but they do not challenge the devaluation of women with mental illness or the very ideology of a marriage "market" that puts price tags on people's productive and reproductive capacities.

Women are not the only ones who experience double binds and exclusion in intimate relations. While men in China are typically expected to be the primary breadwinners in marriages, many male patients I have encountered are kept away from work by pharmaceutical side effects, by family members who insist that they stay home to avoid stress and take their medication, or by employers with no qualms about discriminating against them. As a result, they often feel ignored and looked down upon by their spouses and others around them. As for male patients who are single, their lack of wealth, along with their mental illness diagnoses, severely disadvantages them in the marriage market, rendering romantic love a mere fantasy in many cases. Meanwhile, compared to their female counterparts, male patients are often thought of as sexually overactive. Their parents often worry that the socially-thwarted drive might make them vulnerable to untoward circumstances, such as wasting money on, or being harmed by, sex workers. Therefore, some parents would prohibit them from going out and would secretly follow them if they did.

These exclusions and restrictions can be suffocating. Shaoqiang, a twenty-seven-year-old man diagnosed with schizophrenia, was living with his single mother who had hospitalized him repeatedly because of his behavioral instability. He had never held a job, and his mother had to work odd jobs such as selling food in the street to concurrently support and look after him. When we spoke at the hospital, Shaoqiang's mother had ended his relationship with a female patient he had met during a prior hospitalization, because the doctor had told her that the couple would produce "freaks." Besides the stigma of mental illness that she had internalized, the mother's intervention also stemmed from her concern that she was too poor to support Shaoqiang's marriage and care for more people with mental illness down the road. After all, in today's China, patrilocal residence is still common, especially among lower-class families (Gruijters and Ermisch 2019), and financial support from the husband's family, especially for newlyweds, is widely expected (Wang 2018).

Frustrated, Shaoqiang handed his mother a knife one day and asked her to cut off his penis. "I have nothing in my life," he said, "and now you don't even allow me to have a friend! I don't want to be a man anymore. Just let me be a woman. I'm controlled (*guan*) everywhere. It's like being in jail all the time." If masculinity in contemporary China entails sexual privileges and social domination, then Shaoqiang's case shows that such privileges are shored up by the intersection of perceived able-bodiedness, access to jobs and wealth, and the predominantly female labor of social reproduction at home. As the medical, discursive, and social treatments around mental illness jeopardize these preconditions, and as the strain on family caregivers makes it difficult for them to support the desired conjugality, the loss of these privileges, and even basic access to intimacy, can make male patients feel emasculated.

Despite the ideological dominance of the nuclear family, scholars of contemporary China have noticed that in trying times, people often turn to more flexible patterns of living, mutual assistance, and family membership across a wider network of kin (Phillips 1993; Whyte 2005). Nevertheless, my fieldwork shows that in the face of SMIs, the kin network is more likely to contract than expand, all the way down to the parent-child—or sometimes even just the mother-child—relation. For instance, Shaoqiang had been diagnosed with schizophrenia in his teens, a few years after his parents' divorce. His father had never paid for child support or his medical expenses, and after the father's sudden death in 2008, the paternal grandparents simply refused to recognize him as their grandchild. His mother had briefly been married to another man, but after learning about Shaoqiang's illness, the man also left her. Since then, even the maternal grandmother had treated Shaoqiang and his mother coldly, accusing the former of being a burden and the latter of foolishly carrying the burden. During my interview, Shaoqing's mother said whenever they needed help, "My neighbors simply shut their doors and ignore us." Still, she blamed herself for their suffering: "It is all my fault. A friend told me that I was doomed. True, I've never been that smart myself."

Many parents of adult patients have shared with me similar experiences of being shunned by other relatives, friends, and neighbors. Avoidance by kin may not be surprising given people's fear of the chronic responsibility for care and what Goffman (1963) called "courtesy stigma," or stigma by association with the patient. Nevertheless, avoidance is an option for some more than others. This is because laws and public opinion strap childrearing responsibilities to parents, especially mothers; because, as in Shaoqiang's mother's last comment, ideas of heredity, fate, and bad choices may all work to frame parents as personally responsible for having produced children with mental illness and as liable for care; and because, as we will discuss later this chapter, proximity to patients, willing or not, may generate empathy and impulse for action.

Of course, parents do not live forever, and this fact brings much anxiety about the future to both parents and patients. Shaoqiang said to me once: "As society moves forward, people like me will surely be abandoned. If Mom is not here, I will not be able to survive. So, I may as well kill myself now." Parents' solutions are usually less dramatic, although occasionally there are reports of parents who, after tirelessly caring for disabled children for decades, have attempted to or successfully killed them so that they will not be left alone (Zhang 2017). Much more often, parents try to entrust or transfer responsibilities of care to other family members. The patients' siblings are an obvious choice, but because of the one-child policy which was effective from 1982 to 2015, many patients simply do not have siblings.[2] Even when they do, the siblings have usually established their own households and are unable or unwilling to care for another person (Peng, Ma, and Ran 2022). Alternatively, some middle-class parents in Nanhua have tried to use their socioeconomic advantages to arrange marriages for the patient so that the spouse can carry on caregiving tasks. After all, marriage is one of the few ways for outsiders to obtain Nanhua's precious household registration status (户口/*hukou*, similar to permanent residency in the United States, but tied to a specific city or town rather than a country), which is a gateway to numerous resources in the affluent coastal city. As we have seen, however, conjugality is ridden with fragilities, and even patients from privileged families are not immune to being ignored, looked down upon, or abandoned by their spouses. Many broken hearts result from such arranged marriages.

Rather than entrusting patients to other people who are not always reliable or even available, some parents choose to commit them in the hospital for the rest of their lives. In those cases, what shapes the parents' decision is not so much the patients' conditions as their own vulnerability.[3] For example, a Mr. Xie told me that since the previous hospitalization twenty-four years before, his son Yang had been doing quite well at home. The only problem was that Yang had recently spent all his pocket money buying fancy shoes, and then dared to ask his father and uncle for more. These small issues had triggered bigger worries for Mr. Xie: because he was already eighty years old and his wife had passed away, he was unsure if he could look after (*guan*) Yang anymore, and nobody else could. The hospital appeared to him to be the inevitable choice.

Besides parents, other family members who perceive themselves as too vulnerable to care may also resort to permanent hospitalization. As Mr. Xie's comment suggests, they typically see hospitalization as a means to *guan*, which is similar to the *guan* they practice at home. In fact, some caregivers see long-term hospitalization as a luxury: either the family must be independently rich, or the patient must have public medical insurance and pensions so that the caregiver can transfer the money to the hospital and have the patient stay there indefinitely. This high price should presumably guarantee good, professional patient care and management services.

Understandably, patients typically perceive lifelong hospitalization as abandonment, especially if their family members have stopped visiting them.

At Benevolence, I met Zhen, a woman who had been living there for eight years. When I asked her what her biggest wish was, she told me in tears, "I really wish I could go home, even just for a holiday meal. We all have a need for family life. You do too, right?" Then she wiped her tears and sighed, "Oh well, I guess I should stay here, because the hospital needs a corpse like mine to advance medical knowledge." "Corpse?" I asked in confusion. It turned out that Zhen's arms had been bruised and scarred by repeated intravenous injections, and every injection had felt like some nurse's trial and error. "But I don't care," Zhen said. "Whenever they try things on me, I just lie there as if I were dead."

Whether in a long-term stay or not, many hospital inpatients feel reduced to physical bodies existing solely for biomedical experiments. Those experiments are not done for their own sake, they believe, but for the production of scientific knowledge and profits. For Zhen and others who are left in the hospital forever, this sense of bare life (Agamben 1998) is entangled with, and intensified by, a sense of social death (Kleinman 2009b)—that is, being permanently segregated from society and losing all meaningful ties. These patients exist as what Biehl (2010) calls "human pharmakons": persons relegated by science and families to "dying at the crux between abandonment and overmedication" (222). In the patients' own words, the constraints that come with institutional measures of *guan* give them the feeling of 不管/ *buguan*—that is, being a person of no concern.[4]

As Pinto (2014) points out, the clear-cut ethical distinctions between the good and the bad, endorsed by global psychiatry, often collapse in human relationships amid mental illness. We see similar tensions and ambiguity in family practices such as the use of indefinite hospitalization. Meanwhile, in his study of community psychiatry in the United States, Paul Brodwin (2012) argues that the tension frontline case managers face in their everyday work is not separate from normative discourses but rather "coproduced by high-order mandates as well as the local context of practice" (15). Indeed, the tension we witness is conditioned by caregivers' vulnerability, by a lack of external support, and by a paradox in psychiatric epistemology and practice: on the one hand, psychiatry uses *guan* to respond to, or even incite, people's intimate concerns and hope for their loved ones; on the other hand, it reconfigures these sentiments not only into chronic responsibility but also into indifferent approaches to its realization. After all, if *guan* is defined as using biomedical measures to care for and manage the perpetually risky patient, then how and where it is practiced is immaterial. Nevertheless, the indifferent measures of *guan* that relegate patients to institutions make them feel that their lives do not matter to anyone anymore, not even to their loved ones, and that they are excluded from the intimate concerns of *guan*.

The Story of "Much Joy"

While ideas of disorder, risk, and chronicity render some existing relationships fragile, new ties may also grow, as people explore new ways of being together and flexible meanings of being "normal." The story of the "much joy" couple is a representative example. In 2013, soon after I started fieldwork at BeWell, a social work center serving both patients and their families in Nanhua, I came to know Uncle Huan (meaning "joy"),[5] a family member in his early sixties. He would often use his ringing voice to gather other clients for entertainment activities outside the center, such as karaoke, lunch/dinner parties, and excursions. No matter where he went, a woman in her mid-thirties named Sister Duo (meaning "much") would quietly follow him.[6] I initially assumed she was Uncle Huan's daughter, because most clients at the center were patients and their parents. It turned out that Sister Duo had indeed long been diagnosed with schizophrenia, but she and Uncle Huan were romantic partners. Quite a few people, especially those who had just gotten to know them, remarked behind their backs: while others were busy getting rid of their mentally ill spouses, why did he want to date a "madwoman"?

I carefully raised this question in an interview with Uncle Huan. Smiling, he told me that compared to his ex-wife, a "normal" woman who was ill-tempered and had regularly hurled verbal abuse at him, he actually preferred a woman with mental illness. "Normally she [Duo] is very kind and quiet. When she throws tantrums, I know that it's only because of her illness, not because of her innate personality. It's easier for me to accept that." In other words, whereas other people might see the patient as a carrier of chronic pathology, he was able to distinguish the person from the pathology, embrace the person, and bracket the pathology. Of course, the kind and quiet core that he discerned in her fit the widely desirable image of docile femininity. Additionally, as a man who had not held a stable job for years since quitting his failing work unit, he might not have many options in the marketplace of intimacy, aside from a woman who had endured discrimination because of her mental illness. Still, people who knew them saw them as having a loving, rather than exploitative, relationship.

Note that Uncle Huan's notion of the "normal" referred not so much to an abstract or universal behavioral norm determined by biomedicine as it referred to what the person was usually like, which could only be known through intimate knowledge and attention. By the time I got to know the "much joy" couple, their relationship had been ongoing for over four years. Uncle Huan could now easily discern Sister Duo's condition and intervene accordingly. Because she usually liked eating at a neighborhood restaurant with him for brunch, her recent refusal to go there suggested that she might have become increasingly troubled by certain thoughts. In situations like this, he would try to keep the pathology under control by reminding her to take her medication on time, slightly adjusting her dosage based on his own experience or the doctor's advice, and ensuring that she took regular naps. If her symptoms continued to escalate, he would consider checking her into an inpatient stay. Such intimate knowledge and attention not only provided the contextual information necessary for biomedical treatment but also helped ensure that the treatment fit the context (Rubinstein 2018) and that it was integrated with other lifestyle adjustments to make for more holistic, fine-grained care.

Besides intermittent unusual behaviors that could be easily demarcated, people diagnosed with SMIs may also have personality quirks and habits that permeate daily life. Instead of changing them to what is considered normal, family members may find it necessary to accommodate these strange ways of being. During my restaurant trips with the couple and other clients at Be-Well, I noticed that Sister Duo always insisted on knowing the price of every item on the menu, finding the cheapest among similar dishes, and using paper and pencil to calculate the total price before allowing other people to order, no matter how long it took. At first, I thought she was trying to prevent overspending. Therefore, when it was my turn to treat the group, I told her there was no need to calculate for me. Uncle Huan gently chimed in: "Let her be. She likes to count. It allows her to concentrate and feel calm." While one might easily diagnose Sister Duo as being compulsive, Uncle Huan's words subtly allowed room for her eccentricities, incorporating them into the couple's—or our common—lifeworld.

Beyond simple accommodation, sometimes people feel the need to take on elements of their loved one's radical differences. According to Uncle Huan, Sister Duo lived in a world full of gods, ghosts, and spirits: she would stay home all day, staring at the lightbulb and talking to the "light god"; she would ask Uncle Huan not to go out with friends, because the "sky god" had informed her that one of his friends was a mass murderer; or she would go out and have fun herself, following the commands of the "sun god" or the "brick god." Uncle Huan would not dismiss the existence of these entities in front of her, even though he knew that they were her delusions. To prevent them from overwhelming her, he endeavored to distract her with various fun activities, which explained why he was so keen on organizing group gatherings. To invite her *out*, he had to walk *into* her enchanted world himself. "Hmm, interesting, the sky god told me the exact opposite," Uncle Huan would say to her. Or "you know what? I am your guardian god. I won't be harmed or let other people harm you." By constructing these "shared delusions" to engage with their loved ones, family members like Uncle Huan embrace differences as shared properties, instead of treating them as symptoms to be eliminated. These practices are similar to those that Karen Nakamura (2013) observed in a community of mutual support for people with schizophrenia in Japan, except that Chinese family members who embrace alterity do so out of intimate knowledge and concern, rather than their own lived experience, without community support or institutional endorsement.

Moreover, Uncle Huan's understanding of Sister Duo's particular conditions, and of mental illness in general, could be said to be biopsychosocial (Nakamura 2013), with psychosocial elements being more fundamental. He articulated his understanding at a caregiver's gathering: "Of course, now that our loved ones have already been put on medication, we have to make sure that they follow through with the regimen. But when the problem had just started, we should have tried to unknot their hearts (解开心结/*jiekai xinjie*)." He explained the knot in Sister Duo's heart using the Maoist language of "thought struggle":[7] "We normal people also have different thoughts fighting each other in our heads. She simply treats them as different spirits [coming from outside telling her what to do]." Although he could not travel back in time to fix whatever had started her thought struggles and knotted them together, this psychosocial understanding allowed him to see her differences through the lens of common humanity and to accept the pathological as part of the ordinary. Through all these interactions with, and understandings of, Sister Duo, Uncle Huan redrew and traversed the normal/pathological divide, embraced her as a relatable, loveable person, and used diverse means—including biomedicine—to construct a world habitable for them both.

Identity, Alterity, and Gendered Practices of Relatedness

The "much joy" couple might be special, for Uncle Huan had openly chosen to be with a person diagnosed with SMI and had willingly dedicated himself to her care. Regardless, I encountered many other caregivers who used diverse relational practices to experiment with various visions of normalcy, personhood, and kinship imaginary.

Oftentimes, caregivers are attached to a normal/pathological divide influenced by both biomedical knowledge and their intimate familiarity with, and expectations of, their loved ones. While psychiatric pathology seems to have taken away the persons they know, bringing them a deep sense of loss, an occasional glimpse of patients' familiar personalities would provide them with much consolation. Aunt Ai, another caregiver I met at Be-Well, often complained with teary eyes about all the mess that her mentally ill son had made, both within and outside the home. Yet one day after the 2014 Spring Festival, she insisted on showing me pictures on her cell phone that her son had taken during their holiday trip, some featuring her. Her broad smile, both in the pictures and in person, bespoke her joy in regaining her once vivacious and lovely son, albeit momentarily. Besides their familiar personalities, patients' small gestures of care, such as telling their family members to wear a coat on a cold day, are often enough to overjoy the latter. In the case of persons with cognitive disabilities, scholars have discovered that their undimmed capacities to care, to empathize, and to hold intimate others in personhood through daily activities give caregivers reasons and rewards for care (de la Luz Ibarra 2010; Taylor 2008). This is also true for persons diagnosed with SMIs and their families.

It is not always possible to find familiarity in patients, for madness may expose one to alterity, or "strangeness which cannot be suppressed" (Levinas 1988, 179). As Emmanuel Levinas argues, it is concerns for the other's alterity and vulnerability that drive one to engage with, and suffer for, the other. In the context of SMI, how alterity is engaged varies from case to case. Sometimes, caregivers try to bring alterity into their own framework of comprehension, as in Uncle Huan's likening of Sister Duo's hallucinations to "thought struggles." Sometimes, the alterity that patients display does not allow for even tentative comprehension, but only companionship or copresence in their situations.

Copresence may be built by speaking to patients and enregistering oneself in their terms, as in Uncle Huan's effort to speak to/in Sister Duo's enchanted world. Copresence may be built through listening, even if what one hears "persistently disrupts the security of what is known for sure" (Stevenson 2014, 2). Lina, an architect in her thirties, felt that she was having sex with an Italian soccer star several times a day. Although she lived alone, she called her mother every evening to share vivid details of her experience, an act that initially surprised me given how taboo discussions of sex typically are between Chinese parents and children. Lina told me that she enjoyed the emotional warmth of being listened to. Meanwhile, although Lina's experience was unfamiliar to her, the mother listened attentively, because she appreciated having Lina's trust and the opportunity to learn how Lina was doing every day. In still other cases, copresence may be built through silence. Several patients I encountered habitually wandered the streets, sometimes scavenging in garbage bins. Unable or unwilling to keep them at home, their family members would quietly follow them, trying to ensure that they would not run into any danger and even helping to hold the items they would collect. These caregivers embraced the strange thoughts and behaviors of their loved ones, regardless of their pathological status. Instead of seeing them as risks and striving to eliminate them, these caregivers tried to create safe spaces for the alterities. In so doing, they participated in the lifeworlds of their loved ones and allowed the latter to participate in theirs, thereby building kin relations similar to what Marshall Sahlins (2011) has called the "mutuality of being" (2).

The different ways of relating to patients largely follow a gendered pattern that many of my interlocutors would readily recognize, and deviation from this pattern was partly what made Uncle Huan's story surprising. According to patients and caregivers I interviewed, some fathers have a hard time accepting that their children are ill and in need of support. Their denial may be the result of pride, but it can also become an excuse for them to abscond from their children's care. For instance, Aunt Ai complained that since their son's first hospitalization, her husband had never asked about or gone to see their son. He would get angry whenever she referred to their son in his presence, not to mention bringing the son back home. Furthermore, he had never paid anything for his son's treatment, despite having the only stable income until recently. Other fathers try to beat sense into their children—to restore behavioral and familial order with force. Lina told me that during her chaotic moments, her father had beaten her and forbidden her mother from taking her to the hospital, saying that she was faking it and not thinking straight. Still other fathers are more involved in their children's care, but they tend to emphasize symptom management through medication and hospitalization instead of trying to engage with their children's lifeworlds. Once at a workshop, a social worker asked a group of family caregivers whether they were able to communicate with their loved ones diagnosed with SMIs. All three men present shook their heads, saying that their children were ill-tempered and had no sense. One of them admitted to having nothing to talk to his son about except telling him to take the pills or admonishing him when he became angry. It seems that fathers, and male family members in general, tend to stick to a strict normal/pathological distinction defined by biomedicine, insist on normalizing patients with drugs or coercion, and view patienthood and personhood as at odds with each other. They can also be reluctant to associate themselves with patients' vulnerability and the alterity of madness.

As some of these cases suggest, mothers and other female family members are also invested in the normalizing force of psychiatry. This is because it produces a hope for a cure, however remote, and because it provides a way to manage their loved ones' behaviors that seem disturbing to them. At the same time, they often supplement psychopharmaceuticals with other healing practices such as Chinese medicine or religious healing to address the side effects and help their loved ones gain a more holistic form of wellness (Ma 2012). Like fathers, mothers often grieve for the "normal" and familiar children "lost" to mental illness. However, they are more likely to accept patients' vulnerability and to engage with patients' radically different lifeworlds, even if it means their own vulnerability and life changes.[8] At the aforementioned workshop, most women—though not all—responded to the social worker's question by saying that they could and should communicate with their loved ones who had been diagnosed with SMIs. Some of the strategies they mentioned included waiting for their loved ones to calm down from agitation and apologizing for their own mistakes in a conflict first.

Throughout the long journey to recovery, mothers often act as mediators between vulnerable patients and stern-faced fathers, trying to build a warm and accommodating household with them. According to Aunt Chen, when her son became deranged after working in another city for several years, she had to persuade her proud husband to welcome him back home. Later, when her husband accepted their son's illness but insisted that he stay home and do nothing except take medication, she had to convince her husband to let him work again. "I just wanted him [my son] to try. What if it worked out for him? You know, mothers don't easily give up on their children." When she told me this during an interview, I asked whether these gender differences applied to other parents she knew. "Sure," she said, "mothers are more compassionate (慈/ci) [than fathers]."

In this comment, Aunt Chen invoked a common Chinese saying on parenting: strict fathers, compassionate mothers (严父慈母/yanfu cimu). That is, fathers are supposed to discipline children according to established principles, whereas mothers are expected to be loving, nurturing, and understanding (Kuan 2015). In imperial China, as families and clans valorized paternal authority and male inheritance extending across branches and generations (Fei 1962; Hsu 1971), women had to construct what Margery Wolf

(1972) called "uterine families"—bonds of nurturance and belonging with their children—in order to gain emotional support and to ensure future care. Today, although the extended patrilineal household is rare, public discourse still views mothers as the natural and primary caretakers of their children. In the context of SMIS, because of their everyday proximity, mothers are more likely to be exposed to patients' alterity and vulnerability. As Cary Wolfe (2008) suggests, our "physical exposure to vulnerability and mortality" is connected to "the exposure of our concepts to the confrontation with skepticism" (8). Therefore, it is understandable that mothers' compassionate engagement involves experimenting with and traversing the epistemological and ontological boundaries of normalcy, recognizing patients' personhood and forging kin relations despite radical differences.

"Cripping" the Normative and Normalizing Family

In this chapter, we have seen how the family as a normative ideal and the family as a normalizing institution are mutually reinforcing, harming its subjects and excluding those who do not fit. In the reform era, people tend to imagine romantic love and marriage as a haven from market and social ills available to everyone. Nevertheless, the chronic risk and responsibility that psychiatry highlights in SMIS shows that these normative ties are saturated with market calculations and premised on biomedical normalcy; those who are seen as medically abnormal, hereditarily damaging, and unable to fulfill normative gender roles appear to be bad investments. Thus, they are often excluded from or marginalized in love and marriage. This is especially—though not only—the case for women, as their perceived value lies in biological and social reproduction.

Meanwhile, when faced with SMIS, the family is supposed to take on another normative form—that is, being a paternalistic unit to manage patients' risk of illness progression and to get them closer to biomedical normality. In reality, as we have learned, the family that concerns itself with patients often means the aging parents. Most of them do take the biomedical notion of normalcy seriously, and some—especially fathers—tend to impose it with force, thereby risking the infliction of what Eunjung Kim (2017) has called "curative violence" (14). Moreover, as the ultimate measure of normalization and risk management, some family members decide to have patients hospitalized indefinitely. This measure of *guan* turns out to produce social death, and its indifferent quality fundamentally conflicts with people's—especially patients'—desire for intimate relations inherent in the notion of *guan*. In other words, the paternalistic normalization may harm the very people for which it claims to care.

In other instances, family members may expand and redefine the notion of normalcy to include the person with whom they are familiar, and they may explain the person's differences via the lens of common humanity. These practices allow them to accommodate a wider range of behavior, tailor treatment and everyday interactions to their loved ones' needs, and build a mutually habitable relationship. Family members may even disregard the notion of normalcy altogether and choose to engage with the radically strange lifeworlds of loved ones diagnosed with smis on their own terms. Such expansive, flexible engagement often comes from mothers: they might be too vulnerable to enact the paternalistic normalization; meanwhile, they are typically closer to, and more compassionate toward their loved ones because of the gendered care arrangements. As such, a form of maternal engagement exists alongside the biomedical and paternalistic normalization that is expected of family members but which they are often unable to realize.

So far, we have only seen families' practices of, and challenges to, paternalism in efforts to achieve patients' and their own well-being. In the next chapter, we will explore the enactment of paternalism on the population level and the concatenation of *guan* to the public order.

4

BIOPOLITICAL PATERNALISM AND ITS MATERNAL
SUPPLEMENTS IN COMMUNITY MENTAL HEALTH

In November 2010, the *New York Times* published two articles on the inadequacies of mental health treatment in China. In the first, the authors discussed the "dearth of care" in the Chinese household:

> Left to their own devices, some relatives resort to heartbreaking solutions. In 2007, He Jiyue, a government psychiatrist, discovered a 46-year-old man locked behind a metal door in a stinking room in a rural Hebei Province home. The man was mentally ill, his aged parents told Dr. He. They had locked him up after he attacked his uncle.
>
> That was 28 years earlier. The man, a high school graduate, could no longer speak. "I said to the parents: 'How could you do this to somebody?'" Dr. He recalled. They replied, "We had no choice."
>
> In the past three years, Chinese mental health workers have rescued 339 other people whose relatives were too poor, ignorant or ashamed to seek treatment. Some, shackled in outdoor sheds, were "treated just like animals," said Dr. Liu Jin, of the Peking University Mental Health Institute. (LaFraniere 2010)

The doctors in the previous news article were involved in the "Unlock Action" (解锁行动/*Jiesuo Xingdong*), which sought to eradicate the home confinement of patients diagnosed with SMIs.[1] The action led to a broader national community mental health program—the 686 Program—established by the Ministry of Health in 2004 and promoted in full force since 2010. Aimed at building a nationwide mental health infrastructure that extends beyond psychiatric hospitals and reaches patients living at home, the 686 Program trains general practitioners and nurses to visit patients regularly, monitor their symptoms and risk of violence, and offer them or refer them to necessary treatment. With only a few years' development, the program has become "the world's largest—and arguably the most important—mental health services demonstration project" (Good and Good 2012, 175).

When missionaries established the first asylum for the insane in China more than a century ago, they invoked the image of home confinement to portray their efforts as a humanitarian project that freed the innocent individual from the oppressive patriarchy. In recent times, a similar image has been featured in both international and domestic media reports as a major justification of state-sponsored community mental health interventions.[2] Yet as we have seen in previous chapters, hospital psychiatry in the market reform era has come to view and to configure the family as an ally rather than an enemy, which is supposed to act paternalistically to manage the individual diagnosed with SMI. Why, then, is the establishment of the new community mental health program hinged on the image of mental health workers as heroic rescuers vis-à-vis ignorant family members? If home confinement was mandated by the state in late imperial China, why do some family members engage in it or other practices denounced by the state in the present day?

Family and Community Governance in Reform-Era China

With the demise of socialist work units in the 1990s, the Chinese state needed to find a new axis around which to organize and order the social. Especially in the new millennium, widening wealth disparities and frequent social unrest have preoccupied the state with maintaining social stability (Lee and Zhang 2013), while public crises like SARS have highlighted the importance of reconstructing welfare and health service infrastructure (Mason 2016)—all while continuing economic privatization. Loosely referring to various place-based or group-based networks of people, the notion of "community" provides a space and mechanism for this reorganization by dispersing the sites and proliferating the agents of governance, thereby reaching deep into everyday life (Bray 2006; Tomba 2014; Zhang 2012). In community governance, the subjects are no longer "the people"—a unified proletariat citizenry of the socialist state. Rather, they are "the population"—a multiplicity of individuals who exist biologically and who need to be regulated to achieve an "optimal public."[3] Note that while community governance typically happens "at a distance" (Ong and Zhang 2008), it does not reduce the effect of the state. This is because, unlike their counterparts in advanced liberal societies (Rose and Miller 1992), many community programs in China are designed, supervised, or at least partially funded by government institutions (Heberer and Göbel 2011; Read 2012).

Given families' ideological and practical significance in reform-era China, they may figure prominently in community governance. Because the family can be viewed either as a pristine private realm or as a basic social institution, its flexible positioning enables "the continual definition and redefinition of what is within the competence of the state and what is not" (Foucault 1991, 103). Moreover, community governance often entails various constructs of the subject and various techniques of power, ranging from expecting self-responsible individuals to manage themselves to disciplining intractable ones through coercive and carceral means (Rose 1996). As community agents and experts teach family members to interact with one another in specific ways, and as they publicize certain family practices while keeping others private, they are reshaping the image and reality of the state in relation to its citizenry.

This chapter examines how the discourse and practice of China's emerging community mental health apparatus conceptualizes, mobilizes, and molds the family. I do this by tracing the "kinship correlates"—systematic "understandings [and practices] about kinship, marriage, family, and relatedness [that] organize, inform, and naturalize what will count as the nation and citizenship" (McKinnon and Cannell 2013, 24)—undergirding the country's community mental health governance. My fieldwork shows that as community mental health struggles between care, management, and coercion in governing people diagnosed with SMIs, two kinship correlates work in tandem, one of which being biopolitical paternalism. By exposing and intervening into home confinement as well as providing basic biomedical services to the general patient population, the 686 Program presents the state as a father caring for its vulnerable children. Meanwhile, the program portrays these same vulnerable patients as carriers of medical and security risks, and it demands that family members manage them. It equates care with risk management, registers both in terms of *guan,* and assumes that caregivers can smoothly enact their familial paternalistic power to command patients' compliance. Therefore, while it is more clearly articulated in the mental health legislative debates, biopolitical paternalism as a kinship correlate is also formulated in community mental health. This is seen in the interplay between the state's invocation of the paternalistic tradition to construct new public responsibilities for population management and its simultaneous privatization of that management through the outsourcing of care to families.

In what follows, I interrogate the workings of biopolitical paternalism before turning to another kinship correlate of the 686 Program—the ways in which families supplement the program's biopolitical paternalism through compassionate practices coded as maternal and carried out mostly by women. These practices reveal the limits of medicalized care and the hidden edge of psychiatric coercion. Note that the gender ascriptions of the kinship correlates come from both socially constituted roles performed by different groups of people and symbolic representations of masculine, feminine, or other qualities invoked by normative concepts and reinforced by social institutions, even when they are not tied to a particular group (Scott 1999). In particular, while most caregivers are women, men—typically aging fathers—sometimes become primary caregivers, especially when people diagnosed with SMIS have no other living relatives. Because of their unusually high involvement in care, these men would be characterized as "being a father *and* mother" for patients, and they can indeed act maternally, as demonstrated in this chapter.

Community Mental Health and the Formation of Biopolitical Paternalism

The Iron Cage and the Father State

As the previous chapters have shown, while mental health care in the Maoist era was eclectic and community-based, it has become predominantly biomedical and institutional in the reform era since the 1980s. With the retreat of public welfare, families have become the main payers for psychiatric services. Many psychiatrists I interviewed expressed frustration with the concentration of mental health care in a limited number of institutions, because they saw most families as having little knowledge of or access to them. This violated the profession's ethical vision to "serve the people"—a legacy of socialist paternalism. Yan Jun, former director of the mental health division of the Ministry of Health and a key designer of the 686 Program, told me, "Community mental health is a long-cherished hope of psychiatrists from the older generation [who were trained prior to the market reform]."

A golden opportunity for change emerged in the wake of the SARS epidemic in 2003. The inability of hospitals and health departments to handle the outbreak resulted in lost lives, wealth, and public trust, clarifying to the state that public health was crucial for maintaining its priorities of social stability and market productivity. Since then, the government has poured money into constructing a public health system. After years of development, this system now consists of a network of community health stations staffed by general practitioners and nurses subsidized by municipal governments to provide basic public health services. This renewed interest in public health was initially limited to preventing and controlling infectious diseases (Mason 2016). How, then, could psychiatry share the spotlight and insert itself into this new wave of development?

My analysis of media reports and policy documents shows that psychiatrists and allied policymakers turned to the familiar image of home confinement. Like the old version from over a century ago, the new version depicts a crisis of care in which people with mental illness live like animals— wounded, disoriented, smelly, and filthy. However, while the old version saw insane people—men and women alike—as innocent human beings who were only treated like animals by their families, the new version tends to portray them as "savage beasts" (猛兽/mengshou), with violence and danger brought on by mental illness. These individuals, who are mostly male in the new accounts, have reportedly beaten their family members, damaged property, harassed neighbors and villagers, and even committed murder (Cao 2013). Meanwhile, their family members are no longer portrayed as part of oppressive patriarchies but as people who are—in the words of the *New York Times* article cited at the beginning of the chapter—"too poor, ignorant or ashamed to seek treatment," who "had no choice" but to resort to home confinement to tame the "beasts" (LaFraniere 2010). In other words, even though these reports depict home confinement as pure coercion, they view it as an understandable response to patient violence and to families' lack of access to health care.

Psychiatrists and allied policy makers used this tragic image of home confinement to highlight the insufficiency and uneven distribution of mental health resources in China and to call for more government investment. In response, the state found an ideal opportunity to perform care for its citizens while addressing the public outcry against the retreat of welfare and market deprivation. In the mid-2000s, under the banner of the Unlock Action, many local governments sent psychiatrists and officials to discover people with mental illness who had been confined at home. They were freed from the homemade locks, chains, or cages, sent to the psychiatric hospital for treatment, and ideally returned home, recovered. Estimates suggest that the Unlock Action reached thousands of confined individuals nationwide (Guan et al. 2015).

As we can see in figures 4.1 and 4.2, in contemporary reports of home confinement, the family member involved in confining the patient is often an old and weak parent, living with tears and a broken heart. In contrast, state agents leading the unlocking efforts are typically senior male doctors who bring patients held captive in an animal state back to humanity by wielding the miraculous power of biomedicine. For example, in figure 4.3, against the background of a decrepit room and a rusty cage, the doctor appears bright and clean, like

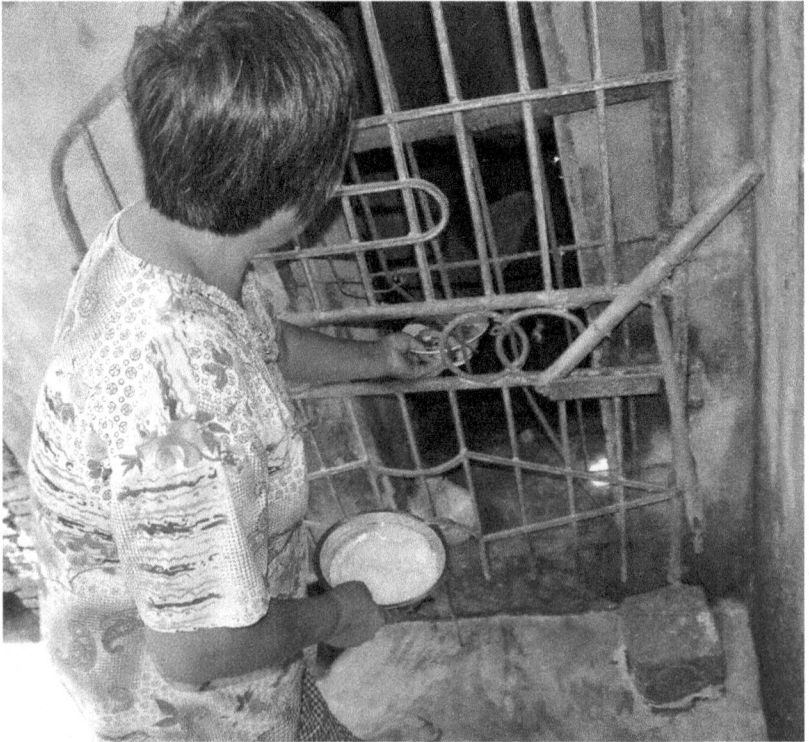

FIGURE 4.1. A man confined in a cage by his parents for twenty-six years.
Source: https://www.sohu.com/picture/300775352. Accessed April 16, 2024.

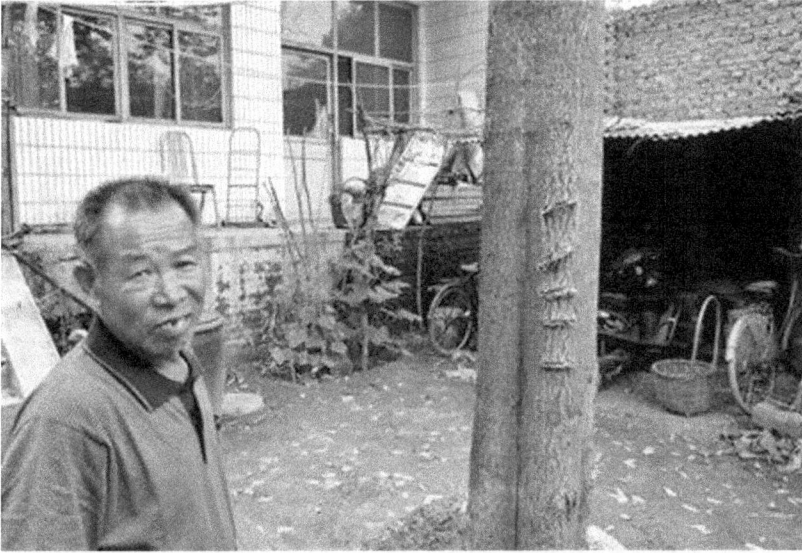

FIGURE 4.2. A father showing the knife wounds his son inflicted on a tree during a psychotic episode. Since then, he has confined his son at home. Photo from Beijing News. Source: http://politics.people.com.cn/n/2013/0711/c1001-22158290.html. Accessed April 16, 2024.

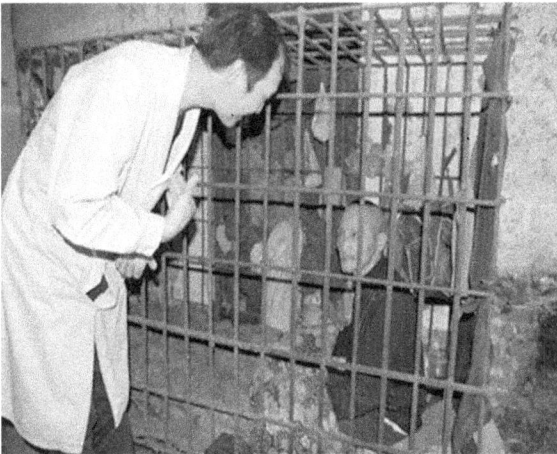

FIGURE 4.3. A man who has lived in a cage for ten years is rescued by hospital psychiatrists. Photo from Beijing News. Source: http://politics.people.com.cn/n/2013/0711/c1001-22158290.html. Accessed April 16, 2024.

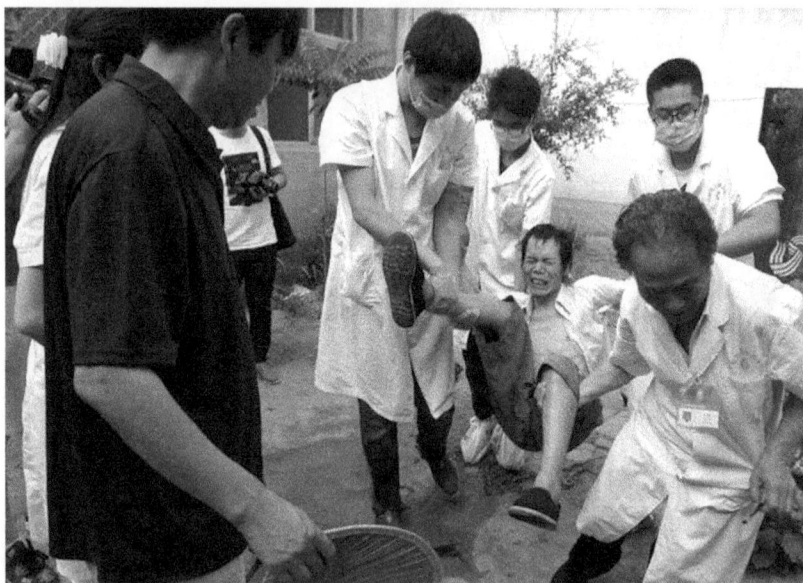

FIGURE 4.4. Doctors carry an unchained man to the hospital while he kicks and screams. Photo from Qilu Net. Source: http://news.hnr.cn/xwgqtj/201606/t20160623 _2550540_9.html. Accessed January 1, 2020.

a beam of light that dispels darkness. His tall but slightly bent body, his smiling face, and the hand gesture accompanying his personal introduction suggest his authority, expertise, and kindness. Upon seeing him, the patient, who it must be assumed had been abject and disoriented, appears lucid and attentive. If the patient resists the unlocking effort, as shown in figure 4.4, then doctors can easily overpower him and take him out of his chaotic lifeworld. In addition, psychiatric treatment can reportedly restore the confined patients' capacity to recognize and relate to their family members—for example, by enabling a chronically mute patient to greet his mother again (Jinan Shenkang Hospital, n.d.). Therefore, while their predecessors at the turn of the twentieth century fashioned themselves against the patriarchal family, contemporary psychiatrists—and the state they represent—appear to embody and enact a set of paternalistic power, knowledge, authority, and care to bring order to the patient and the family.

Besides the "dearth of care," the patient violence that the new image of home confinement highlights is also useful for establishing the community mental health project. By its nature, home confinement is hidden from the outside. The limited number of cases in which it is exposed and eradicated can stand in for an infinite number of (presently or potentially) violent patients who are confined at home or, worse still, roaming free and not managed by anyone.[4] This implication of patient violence makes mental illnesses comparable to infectious diseases, the initial highlight of the state's public health investment: if mobile germs and viruses could kill a large number of people, the mobile person with mental illness could inflict harm on not just their immediate surroundings but also the public. This logic has helped to insert mental health into the growing public health apparatus. Moreover, since the late 1990s, with the rise of socioeconomic inequality and popular unrest, the Chinese state has shown an increasing obsession with monitoring and eliminating any actual or potential threat to its governance or to general social stability. Thus, it now spends the largest proportion of its budget on "stability-maintenance" (*weiwen*) work (Lee and Zhang 2013). Several leading psychiatrists told me that the violent aspect of mental illness had to be highlighted to secure resources from the stability-maintenance apparatus. The image of home confinement provides a potent discursive tool for this purpose. In turn, managing the risk of patient violence has preoccupied the design and operations of community mental health.

Constructing the Paternal Family

The Unlock Action spurred a broader community mental health program in China. In December 2004, the Ministry of Health launched the "Program for Managing and Treating Serious Mental Illnesses, Run by Local [Governments] and Subsidized by the Central [Government]" (中央补助地方严重精神障碍管理治疗项目/*Zhongyang Buzhu Difang Yanzhong Jingshen Zhang'ai Guanli Zhiliao Xiangmu*), also known as the 686 Program, because it was initially funded with RMB 6.86 million (about USD 1 million) in state revenue. The 686 Program's main goals, as stated by its leaders, are "to establish an effective mechanism to comprehensively prevent and control the violent behavior of patients with SMIs; to increase the treatment rate and reduce the violence rate; to disseminate knowledge on mental illness prevention and treatment; and to spread the knowledge of the systematic treatment of SMIs" (Ma et al. 2011, 726). It also defines the scope of SMIs to include schizophrenia, bipolar disorder, schizoaffective disorder, paranoid disorder, epilepsy with psychosis, and intellectual disability with psychosis—all of which have a psychotic component, presumably distort patients' senses of reality, and make them prone to violence (Ministry of Health 2012). Thus, the program connects the prevention and treatment of SMIs or, rather, the management of patients' risk of illness relapse and aggravation to the management of their risk of violence, framing them both as its central mission to *guan*. Thanks to psychiatrists' successful strategy of linking patient management to stability maintenance, government support for the program has steadily increased, and especially since 2010, the program has been aggressively rolled out across the country. In 2015, annual state funding for the 686 Program reached RMB 1.42 billion (about USD 203 million), making it one of China's biggest public health programs (Peking University Sixth Hospital 2016). Most urban and rural communities now have primary care physicians or nurses working as community mental health practitioners (CMHPs) to manage patients.

Before the advent of the 686 Program, psychiatry only endorsed and encouraged the family's paternalistic practices such as involuntary hospitalization to promote the biomedically defined well-being of individual patients. In contrast, the 686 Program fashioned itself as the father state directly caring for individuals in dire need and restoring proper familial authority. Indeed, although the sweeping scale of the Unlock Action has abated, the program still requires CMHPs to watch for cases in which caregivers "lock up or chain" patients "for non-medical purposes," to report these occurrences, and to stop them by sending those patients for free hospital treatment (Ministry of Health 2012). Beyond the Unlock Action, the program's focus has expanded to the larger population of all individuals diagnosed with SMIs, seeking to provide them with services such as free basic psychopharmaceuticals and physical checkups.[5] CMHPs are responsible for connecting them to these services by organizing community clinics with hospital psychiatrists and conducting routine home visits themselves.

Meanwhile, as government support increasingly focuses the 686 Program on patient violence, in the interest of state security, it now also expects and demands families to act paternalistically for the biopolitical task of population management. This task is first delegated to CMHPs, many of whom have said that no matter how hard they work, they are still held accountable—for example, by receiving failing marks on their yearly evaluations—if one patient they manage winds up committing a publicly violent act (Zhu et al. 2018). Even with increased government support, China faces a shortage of CMHPs: one practitioner oversees as many as several hundred patients. Under these circumstances, the 686 Program has come to outsource its care and management tasks back to family members, albeit now with professional state supervision. For instance, in Nanhua, CMHPs typically ask patients' family members—not patients themselves—to visit community clinics to get their medication so that they can supervise intake at home. In their routine home visits, CMHPs usually ask family members about the recent state of patients' conditions, medication compliance, and social functioning. They also solicit family members' reports on recent acts of aggression or violence, which they use to calculate risk level according to the following scale:

LEVEL 0: No behavior listed in Levels 1–5.

LEVEL 1: Verbal threats and screams, but no physical actions.

LEVEL 2: Hitting or smashing nonhuman things, behavior limited to the home, can be stopped by persuasion.

LEVEL 3: Obviously hitting or smashing nonhuman things, regardless of occasion; cannot be stopped by persuasion.

LEVEL 4: Continuous hitting or smashing, regardless of occasion, targeted at objects or human beings; cannot be stopped by persuasion; including self-inflicted injury and suicide.

LEVEL 5: Any violent behavior targeted at human beings, with instruments, arson, or bombing, whether at home or outside.

With a higher risk level comes more frequent visitations and more intense monitoring by CMHPs (Ministry of Health 2012). Note that on this scale, damaging family property only counts as a low-level risk. At the three highest risk levels, the home is not mentioned, except in the most extreme situations.[6] Therefore, instead of treating the home as part of the community that needs to be protected, the 686 Program primarily views the home as a site, and family members as *private* agents, to manage patients' illness and prevent them from harming the *public*. Indeed, home visits typically end with CMHPs exhorting caregivers to monitor or *guan* patients, lest they cause any trouble outside.

The 686 Program sees family members as key to patient management because they can supposedly use their intimate authority, knowledge, and attention to guide patients through medical treatment. As a CMHP told me, "I really like those family members who can urge patients to take the meds and supervise the process. If something happens, they will increase the dosage [based on their own experience or psychiatrists' advice]. Then when the patients get better, they will decrease the dosage." Comments like this are fairly common in CMHPs' public discussions about, and education of, family members. They imagine patients as submissive, easily influenced by their family members. Family members, in turn, are thought to be invested in managing patients solely by psychiatric means through a supposedly open, if hierarchical, relationship, with no coercion or deception on their part needed or warranted. If patients are unwilling to abide by the (medically informed) familial authority, especially when this may lead to illness relapse or a heightened risk of violence, then family members are encouraged to send them to the psychiatric hospital. As such, the family is supposed to act like the paternalistic state and be articulated with its paternalistic institutions, all tasked with and skilled at *guan*.

Covert Medication as a Maternal Supplement

As we have seen, the discourse of community mental health expects and demands family members to act paternalistically, in an authoritative but open fashion, to not only promote patients' biomedical normalcy but also to achieve the biopolitical task of population management. In reality, because caregivers—typically women and aging parents—are often themselves vulnerable, they cannot always count on patients submitting to being managed. Instead, they sometimes must resort to covert, and seemingly coercive, tactics denounced by the program discourse, such as secretly administering medicines to patients (hereafter *covert medication*) or confining patients at home. Interestingly, the CMHPs I encountered often acquiesced to these practices when they would visit patients' homes.

This section and the next will examine these covert and apparently coercive family practices in relation to state agents' reactions. I suggest that these practices allow caregivers to not only act on the state's mandate to manage patients' risk of violence from a vulnerable position but also compassionately prioritize the preservation of patients' well-being, especially their nonmedical desires and lifeworlds. In the previous chapter, we saw how maternal engagement with patients existed alongside the paternalistic normalization that psychiatry expects of family members. Here, drawing on Jacques Derrida's (1997) idea of supplementation, which entails both accretion and substitution, I argue that these maternal practices have come to supplement, rather than merely parallel, the work of biopolitical paternalism in community mental health. On the one hand, they contribute to the mission of patient management, allowing it to work to the fullest extent, beyond existing institutional confines and limited community mental health resources. On the other hand, these practices—especially the everyday labor provided mostly by women, the compassion for suffering they show, and the diverse forms of well-being they enable—offer a maternal alternative to the ideals and demands of biopolitical paternalism. The practical and ontological challenges that these practices pose to biopolitical paternalism render them a "subaltern instance" (Derrida 1997, 145), publicly denounced by the community mental health program, even as it privately relies on them. These covert, seemingly coercive, and ultimately compassionate caregiving practices constitute what I call "maternal supplements" to biopolitical paternalism. The community governance structure reduces them to the supplemental, but their supplemental status in no way renders them insignificant. On the contrary, only by grasping the workings of the supplemental can one understand how the primary—that is, biopolitical paternalism—functions.

A case example illustrates how covert medication works as a maternal supplement. One day in 2014, the CMHP Dr. Xu and I visited the home of a fifty-year-old female patient, Jing. She had been napping in her bedroom while her eighty-year-old mother received us. Dr. Xu asked to check the medications Jing was taking, so the mother went to her own room and fetched a small bottle of perphenazine. In a hushed voice, she told us that every day of the past ten years, she had mixed thirty milligrams of perphenazine with some hepatinica, ground it up, and dissolved the powder into Jing's milk. "I have no choice. My daughter doesn't think she is mentally ill, and she refuses to take any pills. Whenever I ask her to, she just gets mad at me." Like Jing's mother, most caregivers do not hold as much authority as the community mental health discourse assumes they do to win over "noncompliant" patients. Any medical command on their part may incur patients' resistance. Yet they often feel the need to use medication to handle the disruptions that mental illness brings to everyday life, such as Jing's frequent wanderings and occasional yelling at strangers. They also face the pressure—constantly reinforced by CMHPs—to minimize the risks patients pose to others. Thus, covert medication provides a way for these vulnerable caregivers to manage patients while circumventing resistance, protecting themselves, and easing family relations.

Because these female (or elderly) caregivers monitor their loved ones every day, they are intimately exposed to the latter's suffering, desires, and hopes, including those that seem strange from a medical perspective. Thus, covert medication also offers caregivers a way to show compassion for their loved ones and protect their alternative lifeworlds. In Jing's case, her mother told me that she had been diagnosed with schizophrenia in early adulthood. With the goal of calming her down with love and finding a future caregiver for her, the mother had arranged a marriage for her with a large dowry. Unfortunately, it turned out that her husband had been after the money, and he treated her coldly, especially after learning about her diagnosis. Soon after she gave birth to a son, he divorced her and took custody of the child. Since then, Jing had been going to her ex-husband's home every day to try to catch a glimpse of her son, but he did not want to be associated with his "crazy" mother. Jing's mother found it understandable for Jing to resist psychiatric treatment, to hold onto the image—and the self-understanding—of a normal and capable mother. "I can't confront her with her illness," Jing's mother told me, "otherwise it will break her heart."

To simultaneously manage patients and engage compassionately with them, caregivers have to tinker with how to hide pills, similar to the everyday experimentations that parents—especially mothers—of children with other disabilities lovingly conduct (Silverman 2011). It is not rare for these experimentations to falter, to fall short of meeting psychiatric standards. In Jing's case, her psychiatrist had only prescribed her twenty milligrams of perphenazine a day. Her mother had decided to add more, in case she did not finish all the milk. As time passed, Jing's blood pressure rose to dangerously high levels, probably as a result of the long-term overuse of antipsychotics. In some other cases, caregivers do not have the opportunity to hide the pills in food or drinks every day, and fluctuations in medication intake may worsen patients' symptoms. Patients may also suspect, or even uncover, what caregivers are doing and lose trust in them, refusing any food or drink they provide.

Given these compromising qualities, CMHPS *publicly* denounce covert medication. Privately, they often acquiesce and assist with this practice. They may provide caregivers with pills, cooperate with them in front of their loved ones diagnosed with SMIs, or even quietly suggest better ways to hide the pills. In Jing's case, as soon as her mother had finished showing us the pill bottle and put it away, Jing emerged from her bedroom. We all greeted her warmly. Dr. Xu, known to her simply as a community doctor, did not say a word about mental illness. Instead, having gathered from previous visits that she had admitted to having hypertension, the doctor asked her about its symptoms, such as mood swings, dizziness, and sleep problems. She slowly answered the questions with slightly slurred speech. The doctor then told her not to go out so often to avoid falls, and he invited her to the community health station for a checkup. She nodded. As Dr. Xu later told me, the questions and the checkup could reveal not only Jing's hypertension but also the symptoms of schizophrenia and the effects of antipsychotics. At the checkup, he might also be able to prescribe her some antihypertensives, which would serve as a cover for any other pills that she might see her mother handling in the future. Jing's mother recognized the doctor's intention. She beamed on hearing his suggestion and thanked him profusely for his care.

In this way, just as the family's concerns for the patient's well-being, kin relations, and the household's social standing make it complicit in the state's demands for biomedicalized patient management, these requirements make the CMHPS complicit in the family's compassionate practices that nurture their loved ones' nonmedical desires. The concept of supplementation reveals the mutual dependence between the agenda of management in biopolitical paternalism and the practice of compassion in maternal labor. It also reveals the hierarchy and tension between them: while the community mental health discourse, operating on the vision of biopolitical paternalism, openly criticizes caregivers' covert medication practice as secretive and compromising, caregivers quietly push back on having to shoulder the supplemental labor alone when the state turns away. Their appreciation for CMHPS' understanding of, cooperation with, and advice for them shows how they long for the state's recognition and assistance.

The "Problem" of Home Confinement

The 686 Program decries home confinement in even stronger terms than it decries covert medication. After all, its *coercive* appearance contradicts the program's vision of *caring* for the patient—and the public—through pharmaceuticalized risk management. Moreover, the confined patient's reportedly abject, animal-like state constitutes the opposite of the program's ideal of a dignified human. Here, I take inspiration from Yumi Kim's (2022) study of home confinement in turn-of-the-century Japan, which casts a sympathetic look at the practice by situating it in a "domestic and moral economy of caregiving that heavily relied on women's physical and mental labor" (57). Note that while home confinement was endorsed by Japanese law at the time, it is vocally denounced and quietly acknowledged by Chinese practitioners nowadays. As such, the Chinese case offers us a deeper look into the complex state-family dynamics at stake in community mental health and how maternal labor interacts with biopolitical paternalism.

"How Could the Madman Not Be Locked Up?"

My first encounter with home confinement occurred in the summer of 2011. One day, I followed the CMHP Dr. Gao on his home visits to several urbanizing villages on the edges of Nanhua. He brought government-issued bluebooks to record information on each patient in his jurisdiction. One column in the bluebook inquired whether the patient was locked up or chained (关锁/*guansuo*).[7] Not knowing what this meant back then, I asked, "Locked up by the psychiatric hospital?" "No, by the family," Dr. Gao answered.

Driving through rows of glamorous European-style townhouses, we came to Uncle Long's rundown neighborhood. Uncle Long, an eighty-one-year-old man, greeted us warmly and led us to the place where Ah Niu, his mentally ill son, lived. "Just a glance is okay," said Dr. Gao, indicating his familiarity with Ah Niu's condition. Ah Niu was kept in a single-room bungalow that was locked from the outside, with thick iron bars on its only window and no light inside. He was standing near the window, topless and disheveled. Smiling, he greeted Dr. Gao with a "hi." The doctor approached him, gave him a cigarette, and immediately drew back a few feet before asking him how he was doing and whether he was taking any medications. Ah Niu began screaming, and we left the scene.

After this episode, we went to Uncle Long's house nearby. To my surprise, Dr. Gao refused Uncle Long's invitation to enter and instead sat on the doorstep. Uncle Long took out a medley of pill bottles for us to examine. I asked him whether Ah Niu had been willing to take the pills. "Of course not," he responded. "I have to hide them in his rice or soup. And look at the sleeping pills. Whenever I want to go inside and clean his room or change his clothes, I have to mix some of these in his meal and put him to sleep first."

Uncle Long told me he had two other sons and a daughter besides Ah Niu, but they had all married and moved out. Dr. Gao delicately asked whether Uncle Long's wife was still there—she had been paralyzed by a stroke the previous year and, as I learned, the doctor had not gone inside for fear of disturbing her. Uncle Long told us she had passed away earlier in the year, leaving him as his son's sole caregiver.

Ah Niu was now thirty-eight years old and had been ill since 1991. "He used to be the smartest and most filial among all my kids," Uncle Long sighed. In high school, probably in reaction to peer bullying, Ah Niu started having headaches and acting strangely, and doctors later diagnosed him with schizophrenia. He managed to finish school and work for two years, but his symptoms worsened. He began smashing things and hitting people. These behaviors and the repeated hospitalizations—sixteen over the years—made it impossible for him to work anymore. At home, he often screamed in the middle of the night, which drew complaints from neighbors and admonitions from the police. In 2006, his parents decided to lock him up in the room. Unfortunately, even confinement could not contain his aggression. He often threw objects from the window, and he once injured Uncle Long. Over the years, Ah Niu had smashed three CD players that Uncle Long had put in his room. He had also broken the television and the light bulb in the room, which still awaited Uncle Long's repair.

When we were about to leave, Dr. Gao suggested that he might be able to set up a free three-month inpatient stay for Ah Niu, although he was unsure whether the district's quota had been reached that year. Uncle Long shook his head, saying that Ah Niu had been beaten up in the hospital before and would not be willing to return. As we bade Uncle Long goodbye and walked back to the car, Dr. Gao asked me what I had learned from the field so far. "It is the first time I have ever seen a patient locked up," I said, "like those I've seen in the news and as indicated in the bluebook." Dr. Gao raised his voice, with a slightly embarrassed smile: "Oh dear, please don't tell my supervisor that there are patients being locked up here! What you saw does not count; it only counts when the person's hands and feet are tied." I was struck by his definition of confinement, but Dr. Gao shifted gears: "Nowadays people like talking about humanitarianism. Whoever is chained needs to be unchained. But think about Ah Niu. How could he not be locked up?"

In the years of fieldwork following this initial experience, I would encounter three more persons locked up at home, each looked after by women (a mother or wife). Curiously, despite program policies that require CMHPs to report and end the confinement, the CMHPs in all four cases chose not to do so. Two did not raise any concerns at all; the other two (including Dr. Gao) proposed free hospitalization to caregivers but did not insist when they refused. Why? What can the program's public denouncement of home confinement and CMHPs' private acquiescence to it tell us about the workings of biopolitical paternalism? In his equivocation about whether Uncle Long's action constituted confinement, was Dr. Gao acknowledging a different logic of care and kin relations?

The Coercive Edge of Community Mental Health

The discourse of the 686 Program situates home confinement as pure coercion resulting from families' ignorance of, or lack of access to, biomedical care. In reality, the practice is inseparable from the state's focus on risk management, which can go as far as requiring coercion in certain cases. As Dr. Gao had implied, the high risk of violence that Ah Niu posed necessitated his confinement, and the home could serve as a confinement space just as well as the psychiatric hospital. In fact, the home may prove an inevitable choice for most cases, because in the neoliberal market economy, public goods such as free psychiatric beds are scarce. A district-level community mental health supervisor in Nanhua told me that in 2013, her district had more than 4,700 people diagnosed with SMIs but only five free psychiatric beds. Because the aim of the 686 Program is to protect patients from harming the *public*, CMHPs often save these precious resources for patients at or beyond risk Level 3—that is, those who are extremely poor *and* violent and have caused damage or injury *outside* their homes. Patients confined *at* home are typically only able to cause damage or injury within their own households. Therefore, it becomes hard to prioritize free hospitalization for them. Instead, CMHPs provide caregivers with medications to help them subdue the patients at home, ensuring the containment of risk there. By facilitating home confinement, CMHPs are facilitating the biopolitical paternalism of the state, especially the coercive edge of population management,[8] while the state is not even willing to invest sufficient resources into the task of coercion. In this process, the risk caregivers face, especially as women or elderly people handling strong, sometimes aggressive adults, remains unrecognized and even becomes heightened.

Biopolitical paternalism conceals its coercive edge partly by celebrating psychiatry's humanitarian potential and scientific prowess: once moved from the home to the hospital, the patient will supposedly experience miraculous improvement (if not be cured) and will be able to live a dignified human life. Of course, we now know that the public psychiatric beds to which patients confined at home should theoretically be moved may not even exist. Resource shortages aside, the claim of psychiatric efficacy is also questionable. Every individual I have seen confined at home has undergone repeated hospitalizations, and these experiences have disrupted their life trajectories, rendering their recovery and social participation even more precarious. Sometimes, community mental health practitioners privately agree with caregivers that another round of hospitalization would help little. Meanwhile, CMHPs tend to see these cases as among the few that will inevitably degenerate, either because they had not been treated early or systematically enough or because they are simply unlucky. These interpretations uphold psychiatry's discursive supremacy while marking certain patients as irredeemable and as people who should be left at home.

Compassion and the Unbearable Burden of Suffering

When it is available, the free inpatient stay typically lasts only up to three months. Even though it may give them respite, some caregivers hesitate to take the opportunity, in part because they fear patients will retaliate after discharge. In addition to this concern for themselves, these caregivers also fear for patients' feelings and well-being. In my interviews, the caregivers who had chosen to keep patients at home—whether or not they were locked up or in restraints—tended to use the phrase *cannot bear* (不忍/*buren*) to explain their decision. Like Uncle Long, they know from the past that their mentally ill relatives would not only fail to benefit but might well suffer from the inpatient experience. They are troubled by aspects of institutionalization, such as the crowded ward, the physical discomfort, the staff's neglect, potential bullying from other patients, and so on. "My heart ached when I saw him/ her [the patient] go through these," several caregivers told me; "I can't bear seeing him/her suffer again."

The term *cannot bear* has its roots in a gendered history of Chinese thought. According to Mencius, an early sage of Confucianism, humans instinctively cannot bear seeing the suffering of other sentient beings, and such compassion constitutes the starting point of benevolence, a core virtue that undergirds kingly governance (Chen 2007). As Confucianism became institutionalized and adapted into the framework of a gendered and hierarchical order, the ethical sentiment of "cannot bear" or compassion became feminized and devalued. By the twelfth century, "womanly/motherly benevolence" had become associated with the "inability to bear small things" and the "inability to bear [the discomfort resulting from] love/compassion" (Zhu 2013). These associations define the discomfort unbearable to mothers, such as children's growing pains, as minor and necessary costs of realizing greater goals and principles. Therefore, motherly compassion is viewed as a potential weakness that should be reined in by fatherly endurance and discipline.

Today, the historically gendered discourse of "cannot bear" continues to shape different parties' approaches to coercion and compassion. By using the term, caregivers convey their discomfort with the coercive aspect of hospital treatment and the suffering it produces; implicitly, it also constructs their practices at home as less coercive and more compassionate. Meanwhile, especially in public discussions, health professionals often criticize caregivers who express unease with hospitalization as "sentimental," "weak," and "feminine," even when they are men. From the professionals' perspective, the caregivers' womanly (or womanlike) compassion prevents them from seeing how coercion ultimately serves the biomedical vision of care—however remote that is—and the biopolitical task of population management. Therefore, as the maternal labor reveals its compassionate nature and distinguishes itself from psychiatric coercion, biopolitical paternalism discursively disparages it to maintain its own caring image. This occurs despite the fact that in practice, neoliberal social policies rely on caregivers' refusal to choose hospitalization over managing people diagnosed with SMIs at home. Through these entangled readings of "cannot bear," compassion is reinforced as maternal and reduced as a supplement—as a diminished but essential component—of biopolitical paternalism.

Of course, home confinement is not without its burdens. Similar to how confinement of the mad person was integrated into, rather than excluded from, daily household rhythms in Japan (Kim 2022), my fieldwork shows that in Chinese households where patients are locked up, exposure to their suffering is immediate, constant, and substantial. In some cases, the locked room is inside the household and the smells of the patient's unwashed body and excrement permeate the house. In other cases, the patient's room is separated from the main domicile, but family members remain within earshot of the patient's screams and sighs. If caregivers cannot bear the discomfort of letting their loved ones suffer in the hospital, how can they bear the emotional and practical burden of keeping patients at home and witnessing the overwhelming suffering?

The answer is this: these supposedly "sentimentally weak" women (and men) bear the burden through extreme personal effort to alleviate as much of the patient's suffering as possible. Every day, they monitor the patients and send materials into the locked rooms to meet the patients' needs: they serve meals three times a day, often including patients' favorite dishes; they set up water hoses and other cleaning equipment inside the room for patients' sanitation; and as we have seen in Ah Niu's case, they sometimes provide patients with entertainment devices even though the family is living in poverty. These processes of care are fraught, especially because the externally-imposed task of risk containment leaves caregivers to handle patients' potential aggression without public support. Because patients can be calm for a while and suddenly destroy things caregivers take great pains to provide, caregivers regularly adjust the amount of material goods and freedom they feel they should—or can afford to—give patients. Each time they withhold an item or keep a door shut, they regret the contraction of the patient's world while also feeling helpless in having to make that decision. These emotionally and ethically difficult decisions add to the burden quietly borne by caregivers.

As we have learned, in the 686 Program, patients are primarily viewed as sources of potential violence who need to be cured, or at least well-managed, before being recognized as proper humans and reintegrated into society. In contrast, even in the most dire circumstances, caregivers tend to see patients as able to engage and not permanently violent. They strive to connect to patients, monitoring for any signs of kindred recognition, even when patients show aggression or refuse to communicate. In one household, a woman told me that her mentally ill husband had beaten up everyone who had come near his cage, except for his young daughter. In another household, the mother told me that when her son with mental illness once tried to poke her hand with the cigarette she had just given him, she scolded him, threatening not to give him cigarettes anymore. "He stopped, and doesn't do that anymore. What a kid," the mother said with a shrug and a smile. In those moments, at least, caregivers see themselves or other family members as being taken into patients' hearts and participating intrinsically in patients' existence (Sahlins 2011). They interpret changes in patients' behavior, aggressive or otherwise, as emerging from kin relations and expressing kindred affects. This familial and deeply human connection marks the starting point of, and the reward for, caregivers' compassionate engagement.

The suffering that families endure also becomes an emotional burden for CMHPS, but they respond in a different way. When Dr. Gao drew back from Ah Niu's room and refused to enter Uncle Long's house, he apparently felt disturbed by the possibility of seeing the miseries of both the patient behind bars and the mother on her deathbed. Yet his job did not enable him to alleviate the suffering that the neoliberal health and welfare policies had wrought on Long's family. In fact, it probably perpetuated the suffering by demanding that families *guan* or manage patients with high risk of violence through confinement while giving them little support. Meanwhile, in equivocating about whether Uncle Long's arrangements even constituted confinement, he might have tacitly acknowledged an alternative form of *guan* in the household— that is, compassionate care and concern that went beyond the capacity or imagination of community mental health—and that made life more bearable for patients, however slightly. Yet as he turned away from the scenes of suffering, not bearing the burden alongside the caregiver, he shored up the hegemony of the psychiatric, biopolitical vision of *guan*, reinscribing the public image of a powerful, caring father state and the program's mission of population management. Thus, the task of coercion and the practice of compassion were left to the privatized and deprived space called home.[9]

Biopolitical Paternalism and the Politics of Supplementation

As shown in this chapter, community mental health has extended the paternalism at work in psychiatry and attached it flexibly to the state and the family. Using tools such as the revised image of home confinement, the 686 Program defines care biomedically as symptom control and elimination, emphasizing it for the purposes of managing patient violence and maintaining social order as well as registering such care and management in terms of *guan*. This helps fashion the state as a caring father by intervening in home confinement and developing services for the general patient population. Meanwhile, it outsources most responsibilities for *guan* to families, expecting caregivers to embody and smoothly enact a set of paternalistic powers and authority, to have no need for coercion or deception. These processes constitute the work of biopolitical paternalism.

Despite these expectations, caregivers in everyday practice may indeed resort to covert medication and even home confinement. This is partly because as women and elderly individuals, they have to respond to public demands for patient management from a position of vulnerability rather than of paternalistic vigor. Meanwhile, as they listen to patients' cries and sighs, and as they hesitate to discuss the diagnosis with patients, to demand medication compliance, or to seek help through hospitalization, these caregivers also quietly question biopolitical paternalism. They point to its limits of care—in terms of both resource shortages and the inability to address patients' needs—as well as its hidden edge of coercion. By hiding acts of medication and keeping patients at home, they seek to alleviate patients' suffering—including that produced by psychiatric labeling or coercion—and to nourish lifeworlds unrecognized by the biomedical order. Such is a maternal labor of compassion.

To avoid the ethical and ontological challenges posed by these maternal practices, the psychiatric discourse publicly dismisses or decries them as external and counterproductive to the vision of community mental health. In reality, the neoliberal social policies that privatize care and limit the provision of public goods not only treat these practices as acceptable but also render them necessary for risk management and containment. The pressure of *guan* that CMHPS consequently exert on caregivers, as well as the psychopharmaceuticals that the program provides, helps sustain these practices. In Derrida's (1997) terms, caregivers' maternal practices are rendered supplemental to biopolitical paternalism as a "subaltern instance" or even a "negativity of evil" (145). Yet as they "transgress and at the same time respect the interdict" (155) of the primary, these maternal supplements work to fulfill the task of biopolitical paternalism precisely by overcoming its inadequacies and repairing the injuries it causes.

Note that unearthing maternal supplements does not mean glorifying or romanticizing them. The caregivers involved in home confinement or covert medication would be the first to refuse any romanticization. After all, although such practices might make the patient's life a bit more bearable, they are still performed under the pressure of risk management and coercion by the state. Doing supplemental labor when the state turns away also generates much despair and resentment. Still, by considering these supplemental practices with sympathy rather than contempt, we can start to address the problems of biopolitical paternalism. Before doing that, however, we need to know how the work of biopolitical paternalism shapes, and is in turn shaped by, the implementation of the Mental Health Law, as well as caregivers' activism.

5

DETERMINING RISKS AND RESPONSIBILITIES
UNDER THE MENTAL HEALTH LAW

After traveling through the mental health landscape prior to the Mental Health Law (MHL) in the last few chapters, it is time for us to look at how the law has been implemented against this background. We will focus on the law's implementation regarding hospital admission and discharge, the two most controversial areas of psychiatric practice. As we learned in chapter 1, against the scandals of psychiatric abuse, the MHL stipulates the principle of "no risk, no involuntary hospitalization": admission to the psychiatric hospital should be voluntary, except that family members may hospitalize people diagnosed with serious mental illnesses (SMIs) against their will when they pose risks to—or in the law's language, "have the danger to endanger"—themselves and that both family members and the police may do so when patients pose risks to others. Correspondingly, the law declares that patients who are voluntarily admitted may leave the hospital at any time; family members may also discharge the "voluntary patients" and those who are committed because of risks to themselves (National People's Congress 2012).[1]

These stipulations may sound similar to the dangerousness criterion dominating mental health legislations in the United States, which treats individual liberty as a supreme value to safeguard and which requires "a recent overt act, attempt, or threat to inflict substantial harm" to justify involuntary hospitalization (Appelbaum 1994, 27). In China's MHL, however, the concept of risk or "danger to endanger" is undefined and may be subject to a broad range of interpretations. It is also built on existing biomedical and biopolitical configurations of risk, which view any patient as prone to both relapse and violence and which require families to manage such risks in the face of their own precarity. How, then, do people understand, enact, or resist the MHL in relation to these configurations?

From an anthropological perspective, this question is important not because it reveals any "gaps" between the law on paper and the law in practice, as if the former carried the ultimate authority. Rather, it is because people's understanding and enactment of the MHL, as well as their resistance to it, reflect and reshape their everyday experiences of psychiatric care, kin relations, and grassroots management of public safety and biopolitical life. Scholars have pointed out that as institutional sanctions and symbolic constructs, laws can both produce and obscure categories of humans and actions, thereby solidifying or destabilizing cultural hegemony (Lazarus-Black and Hirsch 1994). Meanwhile, laws tend to be abstract and replete with "elasticity, loopholes, malleability" (Nader 1969, 3). As such, people's interpretation, strategic invocation, and circumvention of laws help constitute what they are, and they may in fact bring about surprises. In the words of Elizabeth Davis (2012), law "works metaphorically, asserting ends as if it could produce them, while actually producing effects that do not correspond to those ends" (224). Following these insights, I draw on court cases and everyday applications of the MHL to examine how people struggle to make sense of its abstract and apparently liberal provisions, as well as how these processes open up or foreclose possibilities of actions and relations.[2]

Of particular concern is people's interpretation and determination of risk. As scholars have suggested, risk transforms an uncertain and incalculable future into a seemingly calculable present, calling for actions and interventions (Dean 1998). Yet risk calculation is not merely a technical matter. As Anthony Giddens (1999) reminds us, "there is no risk which can even be described without reference to a value" (5). That is, what kinds of risks are highlighted and how they are calculated depend on the specific ethical values and responsibilities at stake. Accordingly, I examine how risk determination under the MHL is influenced by different sets of responsibilities—such as mandates for intervention and management, liabilities for wrongful hospitalization, and moral duty to care—paying attention to how these responsibilities are distributed across different actors. The co-constituted process of determining risk and deciding responsibilities allows people to renegotiate public/private divides and reorient family relations; they also illuminate the many shades of *guan* in China.

Of course, risk calculations are entangled with not just ethical values but also politico-economic values. As the last several chapters have shown, mental health practices in the market reform era, including their risk management logic, are both products and facilitators of the devolution and selective reemergence of welfare, as well as the reorganization of professional interests. This chapter will further interrogate how MHL practices solidify or rearrange the production and distribution of economic values, such as how the discharge of long-term inpatients might serve or jeopardize psychiatric hospitals' financial interests and how that in turn shapes doctors' views of patients' respective risks. Moreover, risk management is assumed to reduce or eliminate people's vulnerabilities; but because the understanding of risk prioritizes certain ethical and economic values over others and responsibilities for risk containment are distributed unevenly, I also explore whether these processes may elide, aggravate, or create new forms of vulnerabilities.

Negotiating Commitment

The Tragedy of Freedom

On September 10, 2013, an eighty-odd-year-old lady rushed into a district branch of BeWell Family Resource Center, a mental health social work center in Nanhua. She told the staff that her fifty-year-old daughter had long suffered from severe depression with psychosis. Two months earlier, her daughter had stopped taking her medications, become increasingly agitated, and driven her out of their shared apartment. Upon learning this, two social workers visited the patient's home, along with a police officer, a community mental health practitioner (CMHP), an official from the community residents' committee, and the mother.

Because the patient had locked the door from the inside, the group had to break in. They saw the patient naked and restlessly pacing the floor, the whole room sprinkled with some sort of white powder, and belongings tossed about. When asked what was going on, the patient responded impatiently that there was a strange and unpleasant smell. The mother quietly told the group that the "smell" was her hallucination and that she might have used talcum powder to cover it. When the mother suggested that she put on clothes, the latter yelled: "Don't bother (*guan*) me! I'll clean the room myself if it's dirty. Now get out, all of you!"

The group had to retreat outside to discuss intervention strategies. They all agreed that the patient was relapsing and should be sent to a hospital, but the key questions were how and by whom. The MHL stipulates that family members can send a suspected patient to the hospital for diagnosis at any time, whereas the work unit and the police can only do so when the patient is posing a risk to themselves or others.[3] The group agreed that the patient had not endangered others, but did she endanger—or have the potential to endanger—herself so that nonfamily members could step in? What were the criteria to evaluate this? The group could not find an answer.

Fearing potential charges of psychiatric abuse, no one in the group dared to be the first to lay a hand on the patient. Prior to the law, family members could pay to have the psychiatric hospital send a vehicle to "pick up" the patient from home, but the MHL had effectively banned this practice by requiring diagnostic and treatment activities to take place at clinical facilities. The group debated who should provide the vehicle to transport the patient to the hospital. The community police officer present refused to dispatch a police van, claiming that minor trouble at home was not an appropriate reason and that the van could not travel outside of their jurisdiction, not even to the closest psychiatric hospital. The residents' committee official said that the same boundaries applied to their vehicle. Finally, the group agreed that if the patient's mother could find a taxi, they would all force the patient into the vehicle so that no single party would be liable for any wrongdoing. The mother called a few taxi drivers and offered them extra tips to come, but upon hearing that they had to take a psychotic woman to a psychiatric hospital, they all turned down the job.

After failing to reach a solution, the group dispersed and everyone felt helpless. Three days later was the Mid-Autumn Festival, a traditional Chinese holiday in which families often get together. That day, the social workers visited the patient's home again, hoping to check on her and give her a gift basket to establish rapport. The patient did not answer the door, so they left. While walking down the stairs, they heard a loud crash and then people screaming: the patient had just jumped out of the window and killed herself.

I learned of this tragedy two weeks afterward in a meeting called "How to assist patients with SMIs in communities to access involuntary hospitalization and appropriate treatment." The meeting had been organized by social workers at BeWell. Participants included everyone present at the last two visits to the patient, myself, and Dr. Jin, a senior psychiatrist in charge of community mental health at the provincial level. The famed human rights lawyer Huang Xuetao attended via video chat.

The atmosphere at the meeting was somber. Everyone was frowning, and the room was filled with constant sighs. Ken, a senior social worker who had visited the deceased patient, started the meeting. He compared this tragic incident with a previous case in which a female client with whom he had worked also had a sudden behavioral change. Because it was before the MHL had taken effect, he called a hospital van to transport her to the hospital, and the timely intervention, according to him, had improved her condition, allowing her to return home for the holiday. Ken attributed the two cases' different outcomes solely to the law, while downplaying other divergences between them. For example, the woman who killed herself had not received any services from the social workers before the final visits, and therefore did not trust them. This selective comparison implied that the only options available for a patient in crisis were either tragic and dangerous freedom or coercive hospitalization and that the legal language of risk, by prioritizing freedom, made professional interventions impossible.

Lily, a junior social worker also involved in the suicide case, complained that the MHL not only harmed patients but also imposed heavy responsibilities and impossible demands on family members. She recalled the incident with teary eyes and a shaking voice:

> By law, her mother could legally send her [the patient] to the hospital, but her mother was old and frail, while she was big and strong, measuring 1.65 meters tall and weighing 75 kilograms. It was just impossible for her mother to single-handedly restrain her. By law, others might also step in, which we took to mean that a family member had to take the lead. We kept asking the mother to talk the patient into taking her medications or simply put some pills in the water to calm her down, but the mother knew from experience that she was too suspicious to take the pills or drink the water. So what could we do?

Upon hearing the social workers' attack on the liberal-looking law, which she had praised as historic progress (Wu 2016), Huang Xuetao spoke up and suggested a solution that could presumably also protect patient autonomy: advance directives. Signed with a lawyer, a person could designate two trusted individuals to consent to treatment on their behalf in a crisis, provided that the two were of the same opinion. Dr. Jin interjected, pointing out that the MHL did not have any provision for advance directives, and it would not be revised any time soon. He also contended that a judge would not have the professional knowledge to decide if an advance directive had been made with a sound mind or when the supporters could intervene, whereas having a psychiatrist decide would reinforce the medical authority, thereby frustrating the lawyers.[4] Therefore, he argued, Huang's suggestion was simply impractical.

After Dr. Jin's comments, complaints resumed about how the MHL's ban on hospital "pick-up service" was complicating professional interventions. Dr. Jin interjected again. Assuming the position of a policymaker, he explained that a hospital was not a law enforcement agency and thus could not deprive individuals of their freedom. Then he asked why the police had not helped, despite being permitted to under the conditions of the MHL in situations of risk. The community police officer involved in the suicide case had to defend himself: "Well, according to the 686 Program, our job is to deal with violent patients who might create public disturbances (肇事肇祸/*zhaoshi zhaohuo*). Our hands are tied when it comes to patients who don't cause much trouble. Even if we did decide to transport those patients, what if they injured themselves during the process of transportation? Who should be liable for the injuries?" Ken followed up to say that it would have been better to use a hospital van, because the doctor aboard could tranquilize the patient and provide necessary treatment to make the trip easier and safer, whereas using a police van would be not only unsafe but also humiliating. Most of the participants agreed with his assessment.

Although this incident had been tragic, my fieldwork suggests that it represents common struggles which occurred during the first few months under the MHL. Aware of the continued media outcry against psychiatric abuse, professionals and community officials were afraid of being held liable for wrongful hospitalization. Therefore, they tended to read the risk criterion stringently, interpreting it as requiring the patient to display actual or imminent danger in order to qualify for involuntary commitment. They also often pointed to the law's emphasis on patient autonomy as a reason for nonintervention. As hospitalization still dominated the landscape of mental health care, it became a formidable task for family caregivers to get help committing their loved ones, which in some cases produced tragic neglect.

The Desire to Guan

The professionals' and community officials' unwillingness to facilitate commitment threatened to dismantle the hospital-family circuit that had previously enabled everyday psychiatric practices. In the past, people had regarded the hospital "pick-up service" mainly as a commercial service, but its disappearance under the MHL was taken to symbolize a retreat of the state and its agents. For many family members, the risk criterion of the law also ignored the multiple and often hidden vulnerabilities they and the patients faced. For example, the patient in the suicide tragedy had driven her mother out of their shared home, but that had not counted as risk under the law or at least a strict interpretation of it. Therefore, many family caregivers harangued the law, calling for the state to resume its responsibilities of *guan* by providing medical interventions to patients.

These criticisms are best captured in the following encounter. In July 2014, two doctors from Benevolence Hospital went to BeWell to educate its family caregivers about the MHL. After they explained the law's provisions and prohibitions, a caregiver raised his hand. It was Uncle Gu, a retired lowly Communist Party cadre in his seventies. With a worn shirt and his gray hair bristling, he shared his ordeal in securing help for his daughter: when she first became mentally ill in 2007, she just had slightly unstable emotions, but over time, she started smashing things, shaving her head, and refusing to eat. Her siblings urged her to see a psychiatrist, but she refused. Following a friend's suggestion, Uncle Gu had contacted Benevolence and asked for the "pick-up service." By then, big hospitals like Benevolence were already wary of legal troubles around wrongful hospitalization, and they refused to pick up people who had never been diagnosed or hospitalized before. Uncle Gu then turned to community officials for help, but they all looked the other way. Desperate, he brought home some rope in case he needed to restrain his daughter—a sturdy person who had been practicing martial arts—and drag her to the hospital himself. He became so tensely on guard that he could not sleep at night. To his relief, a friend who was a senior psychiatrist at a smaller hospital gave him a bottle of clozapine and told him to put some in his daughter's food. When his daughter was sedated, the friend had a hospital van pick her up. The treatment seemed to him to have arrived too late for his daughter, however. The drugs that the hospital doctors prescribed were ineffective, and he even had to consent to electroshocks. "The situation was totally the state's fault!" he exclaimed. "Now that the MHL has banned the pick-up service altogether, it fucking blocks every one of our options!"

As other caregivers echoed Uncle Gu's complaint, one of the doctors tried to appease the audience by suggesting that the police could help send an at-risk patient for diagnosis. A caregiver said that it was difficult to demonstrate patients' risks to the police, because they were often smart enough to hide their behavior in front of outsiders. Uncle Gu chimed in, saying that the mandate to show impending risk meant that it would be too late for people to call the police. With a raised voice and a reddened face, he continued:

I'll be frank. President Xi Jinping has asked us to build a public service-oriented society (服务型社会/*fuwuxing shehui*). Are we really oriented to public service? No, absolutely not! What is real public service? It should be actively provided [to us, instead of having us beg for it].

Now the law says that oh, we can't seize the patients because many [normal] people have been wronged [by hospitalization]. Have the lawmakers counted what percent of the inpatients have been wronged? You can't let a few cases decide the law! And how can people be wronged anyway? The hospital can evaluate [the patients], and the state can act accordingly . . . The state has many ways to solve the problem, but now the MHL has allowed the public sector to do nothing!

In this quote, Uncle Gu has imagined "the state" as an omniscient and omnipotent agent, which can and should always do good for vulnerable people. Speaking as a person well versed and highly invested in the Party ideology, he continued:

The MHL's principle is highly problematic. It says that we need to respect patients' personal freedom except when they pose risk. Goddamn American-style freedom! Why don't you try crossing the street freely? Human beings are always under control; only control can protect your freedom. Now the whole world is democratic, but does that actually work? That's just fake freedom! Chinese socialism is a sharp contrast to that, and it is real freedom.

Because the patient is already controlled by the mental illness, what we need to manage (*guan*) is the illness, not the person. We manage the illness to protect the person. That's basic logic! Now the MHL says that patients should be able to go in and out of the hospital freely. Great, I guess people [doctors, police, community officials, and so on] just don't need to be concerned with (*guan*) patients anymore, and we just let our society disintegrate.

On the one hand, Uncle Gu sounded like the leading psychiatrists who had drafted the MHL, because they all viewed mental illness as something needing to be managed and socialist paternalism as superior to capitalist freedom. On the other hand, while the leading psychiatrists remained vague about where the paternalistic responsibilities should lie, in effect relegating most responsibilities to patients' families, Uncle Gu unequivocally assigned the responsibilities to the state and its various agents. In other words, for Uncle Gu and other family caregivers who echoed his opinion, the state should provide *guan* to people with mental illness in the form of medication and institutionalization; whether the state and its agents were willing to practice such *guan* would indicate the cohesion of the socialist body politic.

As the caregivers' complaints about the MHL intensified, the two psychiatrists found an excuse to leave the meeting. Later they told me that they mostly agreed with the complaints, but as lowly professionals, they could do nothing to change the situation. In the law's first days, there had been a consensus among many family members, professionals, and community officials that the state should assume more responsibility for *guan* by continuing to allow and enable involuntary hospitalization. Note, however, that not everyone envisioned the same state and social interventions. During the aforementioned family education event, a woman also raised her hand, saying that mental illness, at least her son's, was the result of social pressure and that she hoped the law could provide more community-based services to comfort and support people like him. The psychiatrists did not respond to her comments, and her voice was soon lost amid others' clamor for easier access to hospitalization.

Of course, there were people better positioned to respond to the call for *guan*. At the suicide case meeting, after speaking as an authoritative policymaker to explain the law's patient autonomy principle, Dr. Jin assumed the role of a seasoned psychiatrist and explored how the law—especially its risk criterion—could be reinterpreted, circumvented, or bent to allow access to involuntary hospitalization. Using the example of the case under discussion, he pointed out that when the team entered the apartment, the woman had not contacted her family for days, was disheveled, and had probably not eaten for a while. He asserted that all of these observations meant that she was unable to take care of herself and was at risk of starving herself to death, which would qualify her for commitment.

According to Dr. Jin, the MHL only provided a broad framework for deciding on commitment, and the details should be worked out in practice. Because a seemingly minor act by a person diagnosed with mental illness could have major consequences, the application of the risk criterion should be loosened to allow for more timely intervention. Some participants were concerned that they might get into trouble if they interpreted the law too loosely. In response, Dr. Jin called for a sense of moral responsibility transcending legal dictates and "selfish" concerns:

Now that this tragedy has happened, it's time for us to stop passing the buck and examine whether we can push ourselves a bit further. There are many legal standards that, when read literally, prescribe no obligations for us whatsoever, but we all know the consequence of not intervening (*guan*).

When I was a junior psychiatrist, I was often dispatched to pick up patients. Nobody said it was our [psychiatrists'] responsibility, but we did it out of our professional passion and compassion for the patient. Now you guys are saying that there are all sorts of problems in using the police van, but do you know that I have also been chased and beaten up by patients when I went to pick them up? Every time we dispatched a car, we were also worried about not having enough staff aboard or accidentally injuring the patient when we put him under restraint. It's difficult all the same!

After appealing to people's moral sensibility, Dr. Jin made some pragmatic recommendations. He said that if everyone from relevant departments of the neighborhood were present and if they acted in concert to force the patient into the vehicle, it would amount to a collective determination that the patient was at risk, which would shield them from liability. He also suggested using the 686 Program's six-level scale (see chapter 4) for risk determination under the MHL to make the latter more concrete, convenient, and grounded in existing policies: "As a CMHP, you need to evaluate a patient's risk level during regular home visits anyway. Why can't you evaluate their risk on the spot [so that people can act based on your evaluation]? Isn't the purpose of our risk evaluation to prevent [dangerous] accidents?" Dr. Jin's suggestion reflects an ethic of *guan*, which requires one to respond to another being's suffering, to go out of one's way to intervene in the more vulnerable life, even at the cost of one's own vulnerability. Meanwhile, by loosening the interpretation of the risk criterion in the MHL, he had reshaped the ethics and power effects of *guan*. As human rights activists envisioned it, and as people commonly understood it, the risk criterion was there to safeguard patient autonomy by marking its boundary. Yet by linking the risk criterion to the existing risk surveillance mechanism, the psychiatrist's proposal might reinforce the security logic at work in community mental health. By calling for the coordination of risk assessment and management across different circumstances and by different agents, Dr. Jin's suggestion could make *guan* as security risk management a more prominent rationale for professionals, officials, and caregivers, as well as a more overwhelming practice for patients.

Dr. Jin's suggestion was soon taken up by professionals and community officials involved in mental health care throughout Nanhua. They had improvised ways to loosen the risk criterion to provide medical interventions while circumventing liability, and some of their improvisations had been routinized or even institutionalized in everyday psychiatric practice. For instance, the municipal Center for Disease Control stipulated that if a CMHP determines a patient's risk level to be at or above 3 on the 0–5 scale, then the police may step in and send the patient to the hospital. Note that Level 3 refers to property damage and that injuries to oneself or others only appear at 4 and 5. As such, the transposition of the community risk surveillance mechanism into practices of risk assessment under the MHL has lowered the hospitalization threshold and increased the latitude of public sector involvement.

On paper, the risk criterion in the law is written in nonmedical language; in practice, psychiatrists in Nanhua have come to use medical information to interpret it and to broaden its coverage. They now commonly interpret risks to self as including failure to meet one's needs for food or clothing, inability to take care of oneself, apparent impairment of health, and perversion of the will.[5] Moreover, having a certificate of psychiatric disability or a history of mental illness is seen as proof of (current) risk. Families can commit patients with these characteristics and ask public sector agents for assistance.

Besides broadening the definition of risk, it is also common for psychiatrists to establish a patient's risk after hospitalization, instead of following the reverse order, as required by the MHL. For example, since the law came into effect, psychiatrists at Benevolence have been required to fill out a risk evaluation form for every patient. The form is brief and most of the items included—suicide, injury to oneself, dangerous behavior, wandering without purpose, falling, and dysphagia—are obviously harmful states. Initially, some psychiatrists would matter-of-factly respond "no" to every item on certain patients' forms. In a regular office discussion on how to improve medical record writing, however, the director of a ward picked up a record on which no risks were indicated and yelled at his subordinates: "How can a newly admitted patient have no risks? On what grounds did we hospitalize her?" The psychiatrist on that case responded that the patient's family had sent her to improve her condition. "Well, that just doesn't work under the new MHL," admonished the director. He continued: "We normal people have risks too, like being run over by a car, so how can a psychiatric patient have no risks? When you have a new patient, just write down some risk—any risk—restrain her physically, and ask the guardian to sign the informed consent. We do this to protect us doctors, and to protect society." From the director's perspective, although risks written on the medical records might be manufactured to shield doctors from liability, they are not empty scribbles. On the contrary, he saw risk as a prevalent quality encompassing everyone, especially people with mental illness. Furthermore, his emphasis on protecting society shows that he was concerned not so much with patients as with their supposed threat to public safety. By perceiving, documenting, and seeking to manage risk in such an expansive yet specific way, this psychiatric reading of risk builds on and contributes to the ongoing attempts to construct what Robert Castel (1991) called a "vast hygienist utopia," a hypersecure life of the body politic "to which nothing happens" (289).

Beyond the aforementioned tactics, professionals may even teach caregivers to implicate patients in risky behaviors. During their home visits, I sometimes heard CMHPs telling desperate caregivers: "Well, if the patient had smashed things, the police would definitely have intervened, right? You could smash something worthless at home and tell the police that it was the patient who did it." Few caregivers would follow such advice and blatantly lie in front of patients for fear of retaliation, but many families did search for the slightest hint of risk in patients' lives and exaggerate it to justify their demands for commitment. For example, when committing his bipolar father, a young man told the psychiatrist that his father had recently bought a kitchen knife and waved it in front of him. Later, when I interviewed the father, he said that he had merely replaced the old knife, and even if he had intended to threaten his son with the knife, it would have been impossible because they did not live together. The point is not who was telling the truth; rather, by requiring caregivers to register their need for hospitalization in the language of risk, the MHL in practice has led to a proliferation of risks reported and perceived by caregivers.[6]

The few existing studies of the MHL's implementation suggest that such maneuvers of broadening the interpretation of risk and manufacturing risk are common throughout China.[7] Thanks to these maneuvers, by the end of 2013, doctors at Benevolence and a few smaller psychiatric hospitals in Nanhua had told me that the number of inpatients had returned to the level prior to the MHL; at least in some districts, the police had become more involved in assisting families during patient commitment, and they tried to minimize the harm the process entailed, such as using handcuffs made with softer materials. Nevertheless, many caregivers still complain about the MHL because the law's implementation varies from case to case and place to place, depending on

the ethical orientations, practical concerns, and flexible adjustments professionals and community officials have or implement. Thus, family caregivers
often feel that they must supplicate the state and its agents for vital hospitalization services for their loved ones. Whether their supplications are heard
depends partly on the goodwill of these agents and partly on their ability to
couch their requests in the legal concept of risk, which now conjoins the
biomedical and security logics of risk management.

Debating Discharge

The Hope for Freedom

As we saw in chapter 3, some family members who felt unable to shoulder
the chronic responsibility for care or felt hopeless for patients' recovery
would choose to put patients in the hospital for extended or indefinite stays.
This phenomenon of long-term hospitalization was largely ignored in the
mental health legislative debates, because human rights activists devoted
most of their energy to challenging wrongful admissions. Interestingly, upon
the promulgation of the MHL, some leading psychiatrists began revealing
this phenomenon to the media. For example, the director of Anding Hospital in Beijing reported that out of the 800 inpatients at the hospital, over
100 were long-term patients, with the longest stay surpassing 25 years. At
another psychiatric hospital in Beijing, it was reported that 180 out of the
300 inpatients wanted to go home, and among them, 150 were considered to
be in stable condition. The main reason they could not go home was the lack
of acceptance by their families and the heavy stigma in their communities
(Zhang 2013a).[8] The psychiatrists chose to bring this hidden phenomenon to
light because they thought and hoped that the liberal-orienting MHL would
give the long-term patients a path to freedom and a means of redress. For
instance, Dr. Lin Yongqiang of Guangdong predicted that 90 percent of the
psychiatric inpatients in the province would be released because they did
not meet the risk criterion for involuntary admission (Chen 2012). Dr. Tang
Hongyu of Beijing suggested that long-term inpatients invoke Article 9 of
the law, which forbids the family from abandoning the patient, and sue their
families for "abandonment" (Zhang 2013a).

At the same time, human rights activists also began tackling long-term
hospitalization by working on Xu Wei's case. As mentioned in the introduc-
tory chapter, Wei was an inpatient in Shanghai who had been struggling
for freedom for thirteen years before finally getting in touch with Huang

Xuetao. Huang connected him to a local attorney who helped him file suit against his guardian—his eldest brother—and the hospital mere days after the MHL took effect, demanding that they stop violating his right to liberty. The court initially refused to take the case, claiming that a psychiatric patient was incapable of litigating (Chen 2016b). The attorney contested, and Wei began sending a petition letter to the court each day. Thanks to this unrelenting pressure, in September 2013, the court reversed its decision and took the case. In the pretrial mediation process, it even sent court officials to ask Wei's mother, another elder brother of his, and his residents' committee, if any of them would like to be his guardian instead and to endorse his discharge. Given the court's involvement, Wei and his supporters saw signs of progress and were hopeful for his imminent release.

The Quagmire of Long-Term Hospitalization

As the activists saw it, Xu Wei's case was a simple human rights violation: Wei was capable of self-determination and daily functioning with little professional intervention. He even had the economic means (savings from past work and disability benefits) to live independently. What he and other people in similar situations needed was only recognition of their legal right to autonomy.

Most psychiatrists I encountered also felt uncomfortable about long-term hospitalization, but the reasons for their discomfort were complex; they had much to do with their sense of professional interest, expertise, and ethics. Firstly, rather than seeing it as a violation of rights, psychiatrists tended to view long-term hospitalization as medically problematic: it was unnecessary for patients whose conditions were stable or in remission, and it would even damage their social functioning by depriving them of opportunities to form meaningful social relations. Thus, some leading psychiatrists publicly expressed sympathy for these patients' suffering (Li 2013). Moreover, many psychiatrists found it frustrating to face the same patients whose conditions they could not change day after day, year after year. In fact, some psychiatrists complained to me that their sense of job satisfaction and career achievement was much lower than that of doctors in other specialties where one could make a difference.

Entangled with these sentiments were economic calculations, which varied across locales and institutions. For leading urban psychiatric hospitals, having many long-term residents meant a low rate of hospital bed turnover. As the director of Beijing Anding Hospital told the press, during 2007–2012, the hospital received 40,000 fewer new patients than it could have because of all the long-term occupancies. The director depicted it as a matter of health disparities: among the sixteen million people with SMIs in China, few could receive the inpatient treatment they needed, while those who did not need it stayed on forever (Zhang 2013b). What he did not mention—and what many other psychiatrists told me—was that the low turnover rate also reduced the hospital's revenue. For patients in the acute phase, doctors could legitimately prescribe expensive brand-name drugs and diagnostic examinations (such as MRI scans). Still hopeful for their loved ones' recovery, family members are often willing to shoulder those costs which exceed the public medical insurance coverage. For example, at Benevolence, doctors would usually recommend a three-month course of inpatient treatment for acute patients. In 2013–2014, the first month of treatment typically cost about CNY 10,000–20,000 (USD 1,500–3,000), and the subsequent months typically cost about CNY 6,000 (USD 900) each. In contrast, long-term inpatients often only require cheap generic drugs and regular lab tests, which are covered by the public medical insurance for those who have it. Any expenses beyond these may generate complaints from families, or they may refuse to pay them. To avoid these troubles, Benevolence staff typically kept the monthly bill for a long-term patient at around CNY 3,000 (USD 460) plus moderate food expenses.

In addition, doctors at some hospitals told me that during the 1990s and 2000s, some families had signed contracts with the hospital, agreeing to pay a lump sum up front—which could be as low as CNY 10,000, or about USD 1,500—as well as have it control the patients' health benefits and part or all of their future pensions, if available, in return for them to stay indefinitely. (Some of the patients were as young as their twenties at the time of these contracts.) In the beginning, the lump sum might have seemed like a decent amount, but it was drying up quickly in the inflationary economy. In some cases, the costs of these patients' upkeep had dragged institutions into debt. Given these economic concerns, doctors and administrators at hospitals with large customer bases tended to feel uneasy with having long-term inpatients or, at least, with having too many of them.

Meanwhile, for rural or peri-urban hospitals without large potential customer bases, payment for long-term inpatients—be it from their families or the public medical insurance—constituted an economic lifeline. In my interviews, staff members from such institutions tended to be more ambivalent about prolonged hospitalization. They did recognize the patients' misery, but instead of advocating for the patients' release and return to community life, they would usually ask the government to subsidize the institution more so that they could provide better services. My brief visit to the hospital where Xu Wei stayed suggested that it was one of such lowly peri-urban hospitals, surviving mainly on the income generated from long-term inpatients.

For the state, there is yet a different set of ethical and politico-economic considerations, as revealed in a presentation by Dr. Yu Xin, director of the Peking University Institute of Mental Health. Speaking on a global mental health panel at an anthropology conference held in Boston in 2015, Dr. Yu took a critical stance toward China's mental health system and pointed to the "longer hospitalization and higher readmission rate" as its preeminent problem. He argued that the reason for this phenomenon was that the Chinese government viewed the provision of publicly funded community-based mental health care as expensive, whereas hospitalization was "cheaper and more secure for patients as well as for society."[9] Of course, the government did invest in mental health care but mostly by building big psychiatric hospitals across the country, in some cases with more beds than what the locale would need. According to Dr. Yu, the government was keen on catching up with Euro-American countries on the number of psychiatric hospital beds per capita. Once built, some of these hospitals would face pressure to fill their beds, for which long-term hospitalization would be a good solution. Taken together, these intricate sentiments, concerns, and calculations might work to shape the outcome of inpatients' struggles for freedom.

Back to the Status Quo?

On April 14, 2015, I was in Chicago waiting online with supporters of Xu Wei from across China for the court's adjudication of his case. I was feeling anxious, for I had met many people like Xu Wei during my fieldwork, some of whom had asked me to help them get out of the hospital. Having failed that myself, I was hoping that the verdict for Wei's case could open a door for them.

At about 5 p.m. Beijing time, the news arrived. Xu Wei had lost the case (see figure 5.1). The verdict documented what had happened during the pretrial investigations and the hearing: the hospital and Wei's two brothers had all emphasized Wei's violent behavior in the past, particularly his fight with his father thirteen years before. Over the past few years, hospital psychiatrists had unwaveringly assessed Wei's risk to be on Level 1 on the 0–5 scale—"making verbal threats or screaming without actual damage to any object or person." Recently, when court officials had tried to find an alternative guardian for Wei, they discovered that his elderly mother had converted

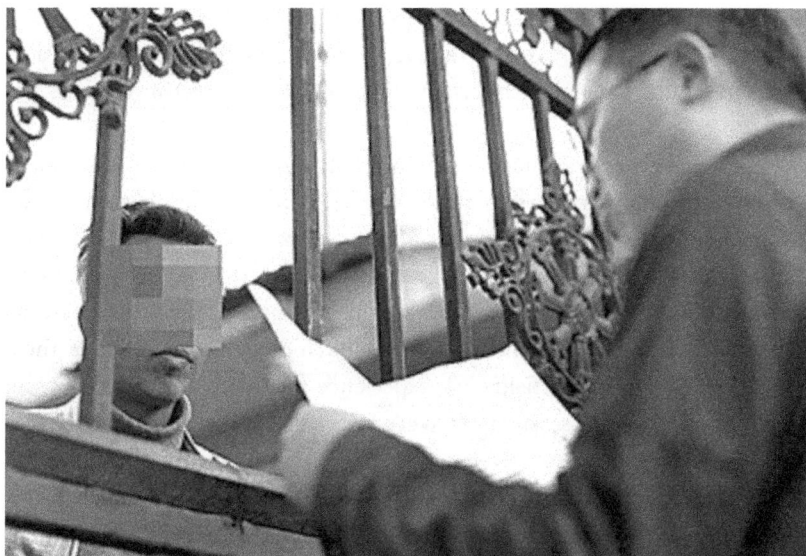

FIGURE 5.1. Attorney reading the verdict of the trial of first instance to Xu Wei at the hospital gate. Photo by Cheung Hing-Yi. Source: https://epaper.gmw.cn/gmrb/html/2015-06/01/nw.D110000gmrb_20150601_1-10.htm. Accessed March 15, 2024.

to a monastic order, his other brother had refused by claiming he was also ill, and officials of his residents' committee had declared their inability to provide one-on-one management (*guan*) to every person diagnosed with mental illness in their jurisdiction. Wei's guardian and eldest brother did not show up to the hearing, but the hospital's attorney defended its decision to keep Wei hospitalized by scaling up the case to a matter of crucial importance to the social order: "There are more than two hundred patients in our hospital and many more throughout Shanghai. If every involuntarily hospitalized patient could file suit and get discharged regardless of their guardian's opinion, that would create a huge problem for the security of the whole society."

After reviewing the case and arguments, the court declared that as a patient with schizophrenia, Wei had limited capacity for civil conduct and should be under constant management (*guan*) regarding his medications and everyday life. His guardian had both the responsibility *and* the right to arrange for such management. Given the family's circumstances, hospitalization was an appropriate means of management, and thus the guardian had *fulfilled* his responsibility by placing him there. The verdict also stated that although the MHL granted voluntarily admitted inpatients the right to request discharge at any time, Wei had been *in*voluntarily hospitalized and therefore could not enjoy this right (Shanghai No. 1 Interm. People's Ct. 2015).

The online group was shocked. The activists were frustrated by the court's assumption that psychiatric patients needed constant management. They also agreed that the risk logic in the MHL had created a loophole the court had exploited in this case: as long as a patient had exhibited risky behavior on one occasion and had been involuntarily committed, they would permanently be viewed as a risk, and their fate would forever be controlled by their guardian. Moreover, my fieldwork experience made me curious about the hospital's consistent assessment of Wei's risk level, because it seemed to have been manufactured retroactively to justify the hospitalization. Whether my suspicion was grounded or not, the fact that Wei's score was much lower than 3, the commonly adopted threshold for involuntary hospitalization, again reveals the extreme flexibility in determining the presence of risk under the MHL.

Leading psychiatrists involved in policymaking were apparently also sympathetic for Xu Wei. Soon after the verdict was announced, Dr. Liu Xiehe, the founding father of the MHL, told the press that Wei had lost the case merely because he had sued the wrong party: he should have sued his guardian for abandonment, not the hospital for violating his personal freedom (Cheng 2015). Those in the online group found this comment ironic. After all, had the court not declared that Wei's guardian had been fulfilling his responsibility all along? As long as the judicial system defined the person diagnosed with mental illness as an object to be managed, it seemed impossible to determine if and when institutionalization would count as responsible management or abandonment. Moreover, if long-term hospitalization was only viewed as a result of *familial* abandonment, there would be no space to question the broader political economy that had allowed total institutions (Goffman 1961) to live on it or to ask what other professional services should be available for patients and their families. Indeed, in Xu Wei's case, it seemed to his supporters that everyone—not just his family—had abandoned him by refusing to care about his desires, happiness, and well-being.

Because of the court's pivot, Huang Xuetao suspected that external political influences had been at play.[10] No one outside the court could confirm this suspicion, but Huang's thoughts reminded me of subtle changes I had observed in some leading psychiatrists' attitudes: even before Wei's trial, those who had initially clamored for the release of long-term inpatients had become increasingly reticent. In June 2014, at a conference in Beijing, I spoke with a leading psychiatrist who had consulted for the Ministry of Health. We had known each other for a while, and he had long advocated for the community inclusion of persons diagnosed with mental illnesses in China. During break time, I asked him whether some of the long-term inpatients could be released and live together in rental apartments, with regular visits from social workers—a desire that a few inpatients had expressed to me. "No way," he retorted. "The government is concerned with protecting society, not the patient. If nothing bad happens with such group homes, that's fine. But if anything went wrong, who would be liable?" Puzzled by his attitude, I mentioned Xu Wei and the inpatients I had met, asking him what one could do for them. "You can't openly help them," he said. "You might do that under the table, but let me tell you, the law's provision about discharge is not going to loosen up."

I am not suggesting that this or any other psychiatrist had been maneuvering behind Xu Wei's case. In fact, this particular psychiatrist might have seen himself as simply describing the state's security obsessions and kindly advising me to play along. He might even have seen the security concerns as constraints on his own work. Nevertheless, by caving in to such constraints and by advising others to follow the status quo, he and like-minded psychiatrists had at least inadvertently reinforced both the security state apparatus and the economic interests of many psychiatric institutions. Under such discursive, political, and economic conditions, the discharge of long-term inpatients en masse has become impossible. A study has shown that as of January 2014, the number of long-term inpatients at a hospital in Guangzhou was, in fact, slightly more than it had been in May 2013 (Luo et al. 2014). When I visited hospitals in Nanhua again in Summer 2015, patients told me that conditions had returned to what they had been like in the old days: nobody educated them about the MHL anymore, and when they mentioned their hopes for discharge, the staff might diagnose them as having a mood swing or a relapse.

Relations of Risk and the Paradox of *Guan*

As we have seen, after the initial confusion and destabilization, admission to and discharge from the psychiatric hospitals under the MHL seems to have reverted to what it had been before: the number of involuntarily hospitalized individuals has not decreased, and most of the long-term inpatients remain behind bars. This does not mean that the MHL has no impact on mental health care. Rather, it has helped people renegotiate the meanings of risk, responsibility, and vulnerability.

Chapter 1 showed that the imagination of personhood in the mental health legislative debates has been shaped by a divide between the biologically normal individual enjoying the right to autonomy and the pathological subject imposed with the right to health. The MHL has entrenched and reworked this divide by allowing different interpretations of risks. On the one hand, a narrow reading of the risk criterion highlights patients' autonomy but also serves as an excuse for professionals and community officials to avoid liability and refuse responsibility for engagement. This can result in tragic neglect of patients and their families. On the other hand, a looser reading of the risk criterion, coupled with tactical manipulations of risk, allows people to assume more responsibility for patient care without fearing liability. Tethering responsibility and risk in this way means that the complex vulnerabilities facing families can only be framed as patients' risks to themselves or to the public, that such risks can only be managed institutionally and biomedically, and that other ways to support patients are sidelined.

Relatedly, the implementation of the MHL has remapped the relationship between various mental health-care stakeholders. Because the law requires people to register their desire to hospitalize patients in the language of risk, it has made people, especially patients' families, more inclined to perceive and present patients as risky subjects. Meanwhile, given the elasticity and changeability in how professionals and bureaucrats—both perceived as state agents—interpret the law, family caregivers have come to see inpatient care as a public good granted at will by state agents, although they are the ones who pay for it or arrange resources to cover it. Thus, they have come to imagine themselves as supplicants to the state (Davis 1993). In turn, many psychiatric hospitals, including those built by the state, continue to run on long-term patient commitment, thereby limiting the development of other forms of care.

Because the MHL allows for multiple readings but ultimately settles for the status quo, a paradox of *guan* that had already been lurking in mental health care has come to the fore, as seen in the contention around Xu Wei's case. On the one hand, according to the MHL and the court's verdict, a person diagnosed with SMI should be subject to *guan* in the sense of constant risk management, and the family should either provide such management directly or secure it from the hospital. So long as the person's biological and security risks are under control, how and where the management transpires should not matter, ethically or legally. On the other hand, as Xu Wei commented during the litigation process,[11] the problem was precisely that nobody wanted to *guan* him—to concern themselves with his happiness and well-being. Underlying this idea of *guan* is a culturally-entrenched ethical imagination. It hinges on intimate affects and relations; it requires the agent of *guan* to take the trouble to attend to the subject's concrete circumstances, needs, and desires; and it seeks to produce hope and make a difference in the subject's life. Note that although this *guan* draws on a kinship imagination, this kind of kinship is generalized and diffused, and it exceeds the boundaries of the actual family to include members of the state and society.

Many people I have interviewed are uncomfortable with the court's verdict in Xu Wei's case and with the claim that long-term hospitalization is an unproblematic practice of *guan*. They also do not think that the fault lies entirely on Wei's family. In other words, *guan* as an indifferent form of risk management at the family's discretion betrays the intimate connections, the shared responsibilities, the spirit of hope, and the production of difference people commonly expect in *guan*. As the medicolegal apparatus of Chinese psychiatry continues to invoke and reconfigure *guan*, and as the tasks of *guan* qua risk management continue to be imposed on families, the multiplicity and contradictions of *guan* may continue to generate ethical unease while also creating political potentials.

6

SUFFERING, SOCIALITY, AND CITIZENSHIP
AMONG FAMILY CAREGIVERS

One day in April 2014, I followed a group of people diagnosed with SMIS and their family caregivers on an excursion organized by a local branch of the BeWell Family Resource Center. Their households were all registered with the municipal government as low-income, and they all lived in a public housing community on the edge of the city. Most households had been impoverished due to the expensive treatment of and everyday provision for patients, and many caregivers had also lost their jobs during state-owned enterprises' (SOES') massive layoffs starting from the 1990s. Sponsored by the local Communist Party, the excursion that day was to visit the graves of revolutionary martyrs. Most participants cared little about the activity, but they were excited about being able to go out and see the city and were happy to receive a free breakfast—a pastry and a small bottle of milk.

The group took the subway to the martyrs' park. Most of them were exempt from subway fares by municipal policies, because they were either disabled or over sixty years old. Sister Qin, a female caregiver in her forties, was caught trying to use her husband's disability certificate to board the subway. When a subway staffer threatened to confiscate the certificate, a social worker came to intervene, saying that she was just confused. The social worker bought a ticket for her but also quietly admonished her not to covet such small gains (贪小便宜/*tan xiao pianyi*) next time. Sister Qin did not say a word, but she blushed and her eyes filled with tears.

Sister Nan, another middle-aged female caregiver, saw the incident from a distance. On the train, she handed Sister Qin some facial tissues, and they started talking about the arrogant and unsympathetic officials they had encountered. Qin told Nan that she was worried about her minimum living guarantee (低保/*dibao*): payment from a family-based, means-tested cash transfer program that was regularly reviewed and approved by one's residents' committee. She said: "Officials in my residents' committee recently insisted that I was able to work. In the means test of my family, they forced me to write down 600 *yuan* [USD 96.8] as my salary and threatened to cancel my *dibao* altogether if I refused, but this 'income' has lowered the amount of *dibao* that we receive. Look at my husband: he doesn't know how to cook, won't shower or take medication without my constant nagging, and were I not there to keep an eye on him, he would just play with water or even the electrical appliances obsessively. How can I leave him to work?!"

Sister Nan, who had also quit working to look after her husband while living on *dibao*, suggested: "Well, next time they ask you to work, you can just tell them, 'As his guardian, I have to look after my husband. What if I didn't watch him and he went crazy? What if he ran out and beat people up or even slashed at strangers? Believe me, the first person he would attack is you!' Or better still, you can take your husband to the residents' committee and tell the officials, 'Alright, I'm going to work. Now *you* look after him.'"

After pondering Nan's suggestion, Qin shook her head. "It won't work. They would say, 'You are his guardian, not us. How can you not look after him?'"

Sociality and Citizenship Struggles among Family Caregivers

In the previous chapters, we have learned that the medicolegal apparatus of psychiatry in contemporary China defines patient care as risk management, legitimates this management as paternalistic intervention from the state, and displaces most of the paternalistic responsibilities onto the patients' families, especially women like Nan and Qin or aging parents. This process is partly achieved through invoking, reconfiguring, and scaling the idea of *guan* and through naturalizing, concealing, and disciplining caregivers' domestic labor. As the figurative community bureaucrat says, "How can you [a wife] not look after (*guan*) him?"

In this chapter, I examine how the Chinese state's economic, social, and health policies marginalize family caregivers; how they experience, express feelings about, and act on this marginalization; and what forms of sociality enable—and are enabled by—such expressions and actions. Anthropologist Paul Rabinow (1996) has pointed out the emergence of "biosociality"—that is, "a circulation network of identity terms," social relationships, and collective actions based on biological and especially genetic conditions (99). Recent scholarship suggests that we not take disorders as self-evident starting points of patients' or caregivers' sociality but rather emphasize "the political and economic context that makes it necessary to organize around illnesses and biomedical facts" (Silverman 2011, 17). Following this insight, I examine the sociopolitical conditions that allow caregivers to identify and associate with each other and the concrete forms of sociality that emerge in this process.

This sociality is most evident in my fieldwork with caregivers who receive services at BeWell. Its social workers organize lectures, workshops, support groups, and cultural and entertainment activities for family caregivers, as well as conduct individual casework. By word of mouth, caregivers learn about BeWell and come to participate in its activities, often also bringing their loved ones diagnosed with mental illness (to whom social workers refer as "persons in recovery" or 康复者/kangfuzhe) to the sheltered workshop attached to it. Over time, caregivers come to know and befriend each other, exchanging informational, emotional, and practical support and organizing social activities outside of—and independent from—the center. Some of them also advocate for issues of common concern by speaking to the agency staff (who are contracted by and report to the local government), the media, and people from all walks of life who come to visit the famed agency, including government officials from Nanhua and elsewhere. Some caregivers even join the Nanhua Association of People with Mental Illnesses and their Families (NAPMIF), which has been tasked by the municipal Disabled Persons' Federation—a semigovernmental organization—to liaise between the government and individuals affected by mental illness. This chapter will focus on how caregivers at BeWell interact with each other, the claims and actions they make both individually and collaboratively, and how existing discourses and institutions facilitate or impede their claims, actions, and interactions.

Of course, family caregivers in China are not the only ones whose domestic labor is naturalized and concealed. Feminist scholars have pointed out that by assuming citizens to be "free, equal, independent individuals," liberalism denies the vulnerability and dependency inherent to the human condition, relegating the support for dependency—such as caring for the chronically disabled—to the private realm (Kittay 1999; Nussbaum 2006). This tendency is exacerbated by the neoliberal devolution of the welfare state (Boris and Klein 2010), because it not only makes people with disabilities and other needs dependent on caregivers but also renders caregivers dependent on, and vulnerable to, the increasingly uncertain provisions from public institutions (Fraser and Gordon 1994). In response, feminist ethicists of care have advocated for "a connection-based equality" (Kittay 1999, 28) or "just care" (Nishida 2022), which recognizes our inherent dependency as human beings and supports more widely distributed caring relationships. Building on this scholarship, this chapter considers how discourses of dependency marginalize caregivers in a context marked by "neoliberalism with 'Chinese characteristics'" (Harvey 2007, 145), and it provides an empirical case of how caregivers pursue political recognition and economic redistribution (Fraser 1997).

Like Nan and Qin, many caregivers had grown up in the Maoist era and worked in socialist work units, such as SOEs, for many years. The socialist state promised to look after them as long as they identified themselves as its working-class subjects and contributed to its revolutionary project (Steinmüller 2015; Walder 1988). This socialist state paternalism was channeled from a Confucian paternalism, which viewed the father and the emperor as the source of life and order (Hsu 1971). In the market reform era, state paternalism is still upheld as an official ideology, and one can see this in how the state invokes *guan*, with all its kinship connotations, to characterize its relationship with the vulnerable population. Nevertheless, market economy and neoliberal policies have eroded the concrete institutional conditions which enable state paternalism, such as the SOEs that provided people with employment and various resources and activities that encompassed their lives (Cho 2013). With this in mind, I examine how family members' identity as abandoned workers intersects with their identity as neglected caregivers to produce a particularly intractable form of marginality, as well as how caregivers mobilize different discourses of paternalism to register their grievances, to traverse the public/private boundaries, and to claim dependency on the state or market agents.

As will be shown in this chapter, caregivers ask the state to recognize their labor in providing paternalistic care and management to patients while also demanding that the state assume/resume its paternalistic responsibilities for patients and themselves. These demands can be viewed as imaginations and enactments of citizenship, if we follow Lauren Berlant's (1999) definition of *citizenship* as people's "experiential, vernacular" understanding of "their relation to state power and social membership" (55). I use the term *paternalistic citizenship* to highlight how caregivers' citizenship claims for themselves and their loved ones are based not just on illness and care, as concepts such as biological or therapeutic citizenship would have it (Nguyen 2005; Petryna 2004), but also on historically entangled and sedimented notions of paternalistic entitlements. Examining the relational assumptions and institutional conditions underlying ideas of paternalism, we will be able to understand the power and limits of these citizenship claims.

Denial of Dependency and the Production of Everyday Defeat

Nan, Qin, and many other caregivers belong to an urban underclass that has emerged in the market reform era. Aged forty and over by the time of my fieldwork, many of them had lost the jobs on which they had counted for the rest of their lives to the large-scale structural adjustment of SOEs from the 1990s to the early 2000s. Whereas their peers may be successful in finding temporary, low-paid jobs or becoming self-employed (Solinger 2006; J. Yang 2015), they have to stay at home to look after their loved ones diagnosed with SMIs. Like Qin, however, they are often classified by policymakers and street-level bureaucrats as capable of working and therefore undeserving of welfare. While low or even nonexistent household income may qualify them for *dibao* at the moment, they live under the constant fear that some petty official might take it away on a whim. Because of this fear of welfare suspension, many caregivers at the public housing community refer to their families as "marginal households" (边缘户/*bianyuan hu*).

Meanwhile, families with a steady income may not be as vulnerable to the caprices of petty bureaucrats, but they have to rely on themselves when facing the challenges of chronic illness and disability. The situation is particularly dire for households that rely solely on the aging parents' retirement pensions to provide for their mentally ill and unemployed offspring. The public pension is usually not much (in Nanhua, the average monthly amount was about CNY 3,000 or USD 450 in 2014), and it appears especially meager in the face of the inflationary economy and chronic medical expenses. Yet this money is enough to disqualify a two- or three-person household for *dibao*, which has a stringent income eligibility. (As of 2014 in Nanhua, a household would only qualify for full entitlement with a monthly income under CNY 600 or USD 90 per person or under CNY 900 or USD 135 for partial entitlement). This phenomenon, commonly called "the old nurturing the disabled" (老养残/*lao yang can*), is prevalent across China, especially among households with persons with psychiatric, intellectual, or developmental disabilities.[1]

Fengxia, a fifty-year-old woman I met at BeWell, was from one such family. Both she and her younger brother had been diagnosed with schizophrenia in early adulthood. They had previously lived on their parents' double salaries and then pensions. Life back then was difficult—her father would wear the same jacket every day until it was worn out—but bearable. Several months before I met Fengxia, however, her father had passed away. The whole family now had to survive on the eighty-year-old mother's three thousand–*yuan* monthly pension. The brother was being hospitalized on a long-term basis because a stroke had rendered him a hemiplegic a few years before. Apart from what was covered by the public medical insurance, his hospitalization still cost the family one thousand five hundred *yuan* per month. Treatment for her mother's hypertension and herniated disk cost another six hundred *yuan*. As a result, Fengxia had to rely on the free basic medications provided by the community mental health program. With limited income and endless medical expenses, the family had plunged into abject poverty. The day I first met her, Fengxia told a social worker that she could no longer afford the subsidized lunch at BeWell, which only cost five *yuan* a day. She told me: "Mother said, now that we are poor, we have to eat less. On this past lunar New Year's Day [while everyone had finished shopping and was celebrating with festive meals at home], my mother and I went to the grocery store to shop for left-over, unfresh vegetables. At one *yuan* per *jin* [0.5 kilo], we bought 3 *jin* of veggies, and used them to survive the first three days of the New Year ... Alas, we in the 'sandwich class' (夹心阶层/*jiaxin jieceng*) are really miserable." By "sandwich class," Fengxia was referring to the family's predicament of being neither poor enough to qualify for *dibao* nor rich enough to live with any comfort.

Terms like *marginal households, sandwich class,* and *the old nurturing the disabled* all denote a status of marginalization by neoliberal economic and welfare policies. They also reveal several assumptions in contemporary China's social policies: on the one hand, all adults are expected to be independent, productive workers contributing to the market economy. Vulnerable individuals are asked to first and foremost depend on their families, taking state welfare only as a supplement and as a last resort. On the other hand, the work that family members do to care for, manage, and provide for their dependents is regarded by the state not as labor to be compensated but as natural and culturally-determined responsibilities that one can and should carry out on top of gainful employment. As such, these neoliberal policies simultaneously uphold individual independence and intrafamilial dependency (Yan 2016) while denying other needs and realities.

These assumptions of (in)dependence have brought daily defeat to individuals diagnosed with smis as well as their family members. In recent years, the state has started issuing small welfare subsidies to people diagnosed with smis, but it has largely left out their caregivers who may also need support. For example, people officially classified as psychiatrically disabled can use their disability certificates to take public transportation for free or at a discounted rate, but their caregivers are not entitled to this benefit, even though running errands for them entails extensive travel. Therefore, caregivers sometimes use the patients' disability certificates on the sly, but risk being caught, as Sister Qin had done in the opening vignette. The admonition she received shows how agents of state-sponsored institutions police with threats and humiliation to inculcate the idea of self-sufficiency in caregivers, to let them know that state resources are off limits for them.

Moreover, because being disabled is the only way to claim dependency on state welfare (Kohrman 2003), caregivers often maneuver to have patients identified as such. During my fieldwork, some caregivers applied for disability certificates on their patients' behalf without their knowledge. To obtain greater welfare benefits, these caregivers would beg the evaluating psychiatrist to classify the patients in a more severe category, and the psychiatrist would usually comply. The patients would be furious when they discovered their documented disability status, for it would bring them social discrimination and government surveillance. In this way, caregivers' attempts to secure welfare resources and ensure family survival might paradoxically jeopardize family relations.

Given the policies' assumption of intrafamilial dependency, people sometimes devise alternative forms of intimacy to avoid state-imposed mutual bondage. In chapter 3, we witnessed the love story of Uncle Huan and Sister Duo, a woman diagnosed with schizophrenia. Even though the couple had been together for over four years, they had no plans to get married, and this generated gossip in a heteronormative social environment. As Uncle Huan explained to me, this was a conscious choice suggested by Sister Duo's parents. When Sister Duo's ex-husband divorced her because of her mental illness, she went home to live with her parents, surviving on their income. In an effort to ease their own economic burden and to ensure Sister Duo's livelihood over the long run, her parents bought her a small two-bedroom apartment. Having her own property allowed her to be registered as a single-person household. Furthermore, having zero household income and being classified in the most severe disability category entitled Sister Duo to *dibao*. Later when she had started dating Uncle Huan, he had been about to retire and receive a pension. While her parents were happy to have someone to love and care for their daughter, they advised them against marriage lest his pension should disqualify her for *dibao*, leaving the two in a form of poverty unrecognized by the government.

Uncle Huan was content with this arrangement. Neither his pension nor Sister Duo's *dibao* was much, but the money did provide a safety net for them and allowed them to enjoy life a little. When they went out for discounted meals or karaoke sessions with friends from BeWell, Uncle Huan often offered to pick up the check, for he saw others' lives as more difficult. Inspired by the couple, several caregivers at BeWell had tried to set up separate households for their children diagnosed with mental illness, but due to the city's skyrocketing real estate prices, this was out of reach for them. Uncle Huan remarked on this during an interview:

> How strange the state's policy is! When children grow up, they should be independent, but their household registrations (户口/*hukou*) are still with their parents. Only when you have property can you have an independent household registration. This is totally unreasonable!
>
> This policy is simply not right. The parents have toiled their entire lives, and they should not be required to provide for their adult children anymore. Now that the state has admitted that people with psychiatric disabilities are unable to work, it should provide for their livelihood.

State Hypocrisy and Righteous Complicity

Uncle Huan's criticism represents the viewpoint of most caregivers I have interviewed. They see the welfare policies that leave the old nurturing the disabled not only as unreasonable demands but also as signs of the Chinese state betraying its past promises. Some aging parents told me that during the 1980s, when the state was promoting the new one-child policy, it had vowed to provide for parents affected by this policy when they aged,[2] especially if their only children were to pass away or become disabled. The state also promised to care for their sick or disabled offspring. At that time, many people believed in this promise, forsaking the folk wisdom of "raising sons for help in old age" (养儿防老/*yang er fang lao*). Three decades later, as the welfare regime has been radically restructured to encourage individualism and intrafamilial dependency, they find the state's promise broken and themselves forgotten. They do not dare to get sick, for they are the only ones their children can count on. When asked what their biggest worry is, they always say: "When I become too old or pass away, who will look after (*guan*) my child?"

Also broken is the state's promise to secure workers' employment and retirement. When these aging caregivers began working at SOEs, they had been under the impression that their livelihoods would be guaranteed forever. Indeed, before the 1990s, although full-time workers had received only moderate wages, their work units typically provided them with comprehensive benefits, some of which also covered their children (Frazier 2005). As part of the structural adjustment of SOEs that began in the early 1990s, however, the state has "socialized" the benefits system run by work units. Under the new system, both the employer and the employee must contribute to benefit pools administered by municipal governments; contributions to social security must last for fifteen years before the employee is qualified for retirement benefits. The tens of millions of workers who lost their jobs around the early 1990s are expected to shoulder the remaining years of premiums with limited government subsidies. Worse still, for those who had left their work units prior to the pension reform, their service records might not even be recognized by local governments, and they would have to pay all fifteen years of premiums themselves to be entitled to social security. At any rate, none of the benefits now cover dependents.

Doubly marginalized as former workers and present caregivers, these family members are cognizant of what scholars have called sovereignty's "organized hypocrisy"—that is, its repeated violations of the "long-standing norms" to which it "pledge[s] adherence" (Diamant 2005, 152). They see state policies as changing quickly and randomly, but somehow always hitting them the hardest. Because of this systematic disadvantage, they may even feel that the state deliberately deceives and harms them. For example, Uncle Huan was among those whose service records at the work unit had been wiped clean overnight by the pension reform. Once at a gathering with other caregivers, he transposed the current pension scheme onto the past and argued that previously, workers had also had a large amount of their salaries deducted by the state for social security purposes.[3] "Now, with the sudden policy change, the state has pocketed our money for nothing," he said, "Policy change can really kill people."

These feelings of deception and harm in turn allow caregivers to claim resources from the state collectively and creatively. During my fieldwork at BeWell, many caregivers went for brief inpatient stays at small private hospitals turned "sanatoriums" (疗养院/liaoyangyuan) on the city's outskirts. There, they could receive some recuperative medical treatment for their chronic ailments, from intravenous infusions to massage therapy. They could also participate in recreational activities with friends, such as mahjong, bowling, and dancing. These sanatoriums typically charged nothing or very little and were popular among caregivers. One day when Uncle Huan was telling several other caregivers about these facilities and inviting them to join him the next time, one asked how there could be such a good deal. Uncle Huan explained that the hospitals simply concocted or exaggerated patients' diagnoses—for example, by documenting a small amount of artery plaque as a clot—so that they could use the extra health insurance reimbursement to cover the costs for patients' room, board, and entertainment. "But isn't that fraud?" asked an interlocutor. Uncle Huan answered: "Well, we've all bought health insurance from the government. Do you know that every year a person can have 400,000 yuan [approximately USD 60,000] of medical expenses reimbursed? You don't know that because the government has deliberately kept it a secret. We're just getting back what we deserve!"

Uncle Huan's words convinced the other caregivers, and they all agreed to join him the next time. From the perspective of the insurance mechanism, Uncle Huan's understanding is erroneous, for 400,000 yuan is the maximum amount an insured person can claim in a year, not what everyone could use in full. Yet for Uncle Huan and other caregivers, the state is deliberately hiding money from them, as evidenced in the difficulties they routinely encounter when trying to claim benefits and entitlements. To get even, they collude to claim public resources for subsistence, pleasure, and life nurturance. In this process, they form what anthropologist Hans Steinmüller (2010) called "communities of complicity," where they regularly engage in officially denigrated practices and selectively reveal or conceal them to outsiders. Though secretive, caregivers in our case are not embarrassed about their practices; instead, they feel righteous.[4] After all, they see themselves as holding the hypocritical neoliberal state to its paternalistic promise—that is, to recognize citizens' contributions to production and reproduction, to allow or even encourage dependency on it, and to run like a family instead of setting up boundaries.

Besides navigating health care and leisure resources together, caregivers also collectively engage in or refrain from certain emotional expressions. As Sara Ahmed (2014) explains, "emotions work to shape the 'surfaces' of individual and collective bodies . . . by aligning subjects with collectives." She urges us to heed "what sticks" in the circulation of emotions and how that affects social transformation. Thus, the elicitation, display, and circulation of emotions among caregivers can reveal the subjectivity expected of them and the sociality they produce.

During my fieldwork, the staff at BeWell and other community mental health agencies often organized workshops to teach caregivers how to support patients and manage their own emotions. At one such workshop, Dr. Jin, a senior psychiatrist in charge of community mental health work for the province, started by asking caregivers if they had felt any emotional pain after learning about their loved ones' conditions or taking on the caregiving responsibilities. A few caregivers responded with feelings of anger, shame, fear, and depression. Dr. Jin said that these emotional pains revealed the sacrifice that caregivers had incurred and that because no one else had such dedication, the family was of utmost importance for patient care and management. Yet he also attributed the negative emotions to caregivers' obsession with patients and their inability to establish proper boundaries, arguing that these attitudes and behaviors might overwhelm the patients, aggravate their symptoms, and exhaust the caregivers. "Don't pay too much attention to patients," he said. "Instead, cultivate their self-esteem and self-reliance so that they can interact with others, find work, and recover their social functions."

Dr. Jin's teaching was typical of the family education workshops. On those occasions, mental health professionals employed or contracted by the state would frame caregivers' emotional pains as responses to seeing their loved ones suffer, which motivate them to care and are necessary costs of such care. Because these emotions are supposedly spontaneous, care work is also supposed to flow naturally from family love, independent of external demands and not in need of compensation. Meanwhile, by framing these emotions as potentially harmful excesses, mental health professionals seek to regulate them with the goal of not only relieving caregivers but also—and more importantly—expediting patients' recovery. Justified as they are, these teachings ignore the structural factors that make patients and caregivers suffer, such as the discriminatory job market that excludes people diagnosed with mental illness. Scholars of China have pointed out that because negative affects are viewed as politically threatening (Sorace 2018), state agents have increasingly come to ask marginalized people to conceive of themselves as embodying deep interiority that can and should be modified by psychological knowledge so that they can be self-reliant subjects who contribute to the market economy (J. Yang 2015). In this case, caregivers are constructed as individual feeling subjects whose emotions should be modulated to produce well-functioning patients and a well-ordered society.

This emotion configuration and subject construction often fails to stick. At the aforementioned workshop, a caregiver sneered at Dr. Jin's elicitation of emotional pains: "What's the point in talking about this? Let's talk about something practical!" Dr. Jin was flustered for a few seconds before returning to his scripted speech. As the workshop progressed, more caregivers lost interest and started chatting with each other. As such, these caregivers at least unconsciously refused to have their feelings—and the responsibility of patient care and management—individualized; some of them even demanded the state's support for them and their loved ones.

It would be inaccurate to assume that caregivers always refuse to express negative emotions, however. In fact, unprompted by professionals, they often share stories of suffering with each other and help each other construct such stories. Once, I sat in on a family support group at BeWell led by a senior social worker named Linda. Ten caregivers participated in the group, most of whom were new to the agency. After being introduced to each other, the participants began telling each other their worries in caring for their loved ones. Linda tried to interrupt, asking them to discuss group rules first, but the side conversations continued, and they soon gravitated toward Aunt Mai's story: after the death of her brother, her sister-in-law had refused to look after, or even live with, their daughter, Yulan, who had bipolar disorder. Because Yulan had nowhere else to go—unmarried adults were not qualified for public housing if their parents had housing and income—Aunt Mai had opened her home and taken on caregiving responsibilities. Her son and daughter-in-law did not appreciate her dedication to someone outside their immediate family, and they especially hated having to share their tiny apartment with the "madwoman." They kept scolding Yulan and giving her the cold shoulder. As a result, her condition worsened, she was no longer able to work, and she was bothering Aunt Mai's grandson in turn. "I am stuck in between," Aunt Mai told us, sobbing. "I feel so depressed at home. Why does life have to be so difficult?"

Linda tried to divert the conversation so that everyone would have a chance to speak. Interestingly, the other participants did not mind listening to Aunt Mai at all. They nodded to echo her experience, asked questions to facilitate her storytelling, and suggested solutions to her predicaments. For example, one asked why Yulan, a college graduate with previous work experience, did not work to support herself. Aunt Mai said that employers always asked her intrusive questions upon seeing her symptomatic behaviors, such as hand tremors produced by antipsychotics. These questions worried her that her cover would be blown and she would be the subject of discrimination, so she had to quit, and the inability to hold a job had made her even more withdrawn. "Alas, your niece's condition didn't start out that serious," a group member remarked to Aunt Mai, "but it has only gradually worsened. If society had given people like her something to do . . ." "If society had given them something to do," Aunt Mai said, "and if the government had given them a place to live so that they didn't have to rely on others, things would have never gotten this bad." Later, when someone asked Aunt Mai why she had not sent her niece to the hospital, she lamented that she had no money. A few participants told her that the residents' committee could sign the patient up for some free basic health insurance. Aunt Mai said in surprise: "I've visited the residents' committee many times and told them my niece's condition, but they've never told me about this policy." "Well, they are not there to serve," yet another participant chimed in, "but to manage (*guan*) you. They will never ask what you need or what they can do for you."

While Dr. Jin saw caregivers' emotions as ultimately responsible for patients' recovery, caregivers in this group attributed the patient's condition and Aunt Mai's suffering to the irresponsible kin, the discriminating public, the lack of welfare support, and the unhelpful government official. In so doing, these caregivers co-constructed a tale of suffering that represented the predicaments they each faced, and such tales were ubiquitous in my fieldwork. In her work on the development of psychotherapy in China, Li Zhang (2020) has discovered the emergence of a "psychosociality" as middle-class people learn to share narratives of feelings in psychological discourses and therapeutic settings. In my research, a sociality based on narratives of suffering also emerges among caregivers, but instead of adopting the new psychological discourses that sideline structural problems, these underclass caregivers invoke an old genre called "speaking bitterness" (诉苦/*suku*), which the Chinese Communist Party developed in the 1940s and promoted throughout the socialist era. Narratives of this genre register people's suffering in the language of class exploitation and social injustice, thereby allowing them to produce "collective identities as members of oppressed groups" (Huang 2014, 586). Born and raised in the socialist era, today's caregivers also frame their suffering in terms of social, political, and economic marginalization, and they fashion themselves as virtuous subjects, shouldering alone a task that should not have been their (own) responsibility. As Aunt Mai explained: "Sure, I don't have to care (*guan*). I can simply drive her [my niece] away. But how can she survive in society? Look at all those miserable people in the street!"

The "speaking bitterness" genre was an emotional device for inducing people's identification with, and participation in, the socialist revolution, as well as their appreciation of the "sweet lives" that the paternalistic state had provided. Stories in this genre often ended with struggles for, and victories of, collective liberation (Zhu 1992). By narrating their suffering, caregivers in our case also explore ways to repair the injuries they and their loved ones have endured, except that today, the injuries are often inflicted by the state. They even invite listeners to bear witness to their injuries and help them seek repair. In the support group meeting, Linda asked the participants whether they would like me, the visiting researcher, to keep their stories secret. Aunt Chen, an active member at BeWell, answered: "I don't think so. We usually don't want our stories to be known, treating them as our privacy, because we are afraid of discrimination. But now that I'm already like this, fallen to the bottom of society, I want the whole world to pay attention to us, to these forgotten people. So, I think Ms. Ma's visit is a great opportunity. I hope she can truthfully represent our situation, and I hope the state and the health department can take it seriously." All the other participants nodded in agreement.

In refusing to treat their suffering experiences as private matters, caregivers traverse the public/private divide that keeps mental illness and its care a private issue, invisible to the public. They also refuse to be individualized feeling subjects whose interiority can only be accessed and shaped by mental health professionals. By narrating their suffering and its social origins together, caregivers fashion a collective identity as marginalized but virtuous citizens, demanding recognition of and redress for their suffering.

Claiming Paternalistic Citizenship

In the conversation with which I began this chapter, Nan and Qin were also constructing a tale of bitterness and seeking redress together. Nan suggested that Qin confront the government with her difficult work of *guan* and its importance for the social order by highlighting the threat that patient violence would pose to government officials and the public. Indeed, in their gatherings, caregivers often discuss how only tragic events of patient violence would attract the government's attention to their suffering. One time at a meeting, when a social worker told some caregivers about an upcoming policy change that might disqualify them for public housing, one of them said: "Nobody cares about (*guan*) us marginalized households, unless more and more people can't stand it and jump off the building! But no, even that won't work. If you die, it's your own business. The government will just wait and collect your bodies." Later, the social worker mentioned that a patient in another city had recently slashed at strangers in public and injured six people, all policemen. To his surprise, several audience members burst out laughing: "Good job! That person is not crazy at all!"

Sociologists Ching Kwan Lee and Yonghong Zhang (2013) have pointed out that as the Chinese state is increasingly preoccupied with "maintaining stability" and has assembled a large institutional apparatus to "buy stability" from its citizenry, citizens have also begun to consciously use instability and disorder as "their bargaining chip" (1488). In our case, caregivers know that patient violence in public has been registered as a source of instability and can serve as their bargaining chip to draw attention and resources from the state. Granted, most caregivers do not think their loved ones are violent or hope that they act as such, but they might feel a sense of revenge to see incidents of violence incite fear in people—especially government officials—and reveal the importance of their hidden work. In times of desperation, some caregivers might even resort to offering gentle reminders themselves, as Nan suggested Qin do. Although Qin shrugged off the advice, a community mental health official told me that a few seniors in her jurisdiction had taken their adult children diagnosed with SMIs to the local government, demanding welfare support in recognition of their patient management work.

When caregivers take patients to government officials and ask them to look after (*guan*) patients, they might not only be seeking compensation for their contribution to biopolitical paternalism but also to have the state assume paternal responsibility, whether the patients are potentially violent or not. As we have seen, Uncle Huan argued that the state should provide for adult patients who are unable to work, and this argument is echoed by most of the caregivers I have encountered. In my interview, Aunt Gu, then Vice Chair of NAPMIF and a patient's mother, emphasized the time-bound nature of family childrearing and the state's duty of parenting: "Before a child reaches eighteen, it's the family's responsibility [to raise them]. But after eighteen, the child is society's citizen, and society has the responsibility to nurture them. I always raise this issue when meeting with leaders from the provincial or municipal government." While Aunt Gu had used the word *society*, her targeted appeal to government leaders reveals that it mostly referred to the state; she expected the state to provide, or assemble resources to nurture, the mentally ill patients—its own citizens-children.

Invoking this idea of state paternalism, family caregivers have expressed many concrete demands, some of which are being met by local governments. After all, in the face of growing social inequality and popular unrest, the state does want to reclaim a populist, paternalistic image of caring for its people (Duckett and Langer 2013). In 1999, the Nanhua Disabled Persons' Federation founded BeWell as a resource center for family caregivers. Before long, caregivers started to tell federation leaders and social workers that there should also be rehabilitation services for their loved ones diagnosed with mental illness. The federation responded by establishing a clubhouse and a sheltered workshop attached to the center, and for many years the sheltered workshop provided its trainees with modest subsidies (about CNY 500 or USD 75 per month as of 2014).[5] Thanks to caregivers' continued advocacy and to examples set by pioneering agencies like BeWell, these services have emerged across Nanhua and in other major Chinese cities.

To solve "the old nurturing the disabled" problem, caregivers in Nanhua—partly through the NAPMIF's leadership—have been asking the provincial and municipal governments to help pay the premiums for social security and public health insurance for all patients and to grant *dibao* entitlements to patients who cannot work, regardless of their family situation or household income. By 2014, the municipal government had been seriously considering the former request. It had also started to provide financial aid for patients' treatment, as well as small amounts of livelihood and care subsidies for patients and their caregivers, respectively. (In 2014, the livelihood subsidies for impoverished people with severe psychiatric disabilities were CNY 600/year, and the care subsidies were CNY 1,200/year.)

As former socialist workers, many caregivers are attached to the idea—and the historical fact—that the state's paternalistic care was administered by work units. Therefore, they also seek to build paternalistic ties between their loved ones and "work units," which are now companies that follow market logic. The most common practice is to help their loved ones participate in "quota scheme employment" (按比例就业/*an bili jiuye*), a government program established across China in the mid-2000s. The program requires businesses and government sectors to employ a quota of persons with disabilities, and it fines those that do not meet this requirement. To avoid paying the fines, many companies have developed a complicit tactic with persons with disabilities and their families: a company lists a person with a disability as an employee, thus meeting one "quota," but that person does not need to come to work; in return, the company pays the person's social security and health insurance premiums for the duration of their "employment." Sometimes, it would also pay that person a salary, the amount of which would be far lower than the local minimum wage. As such, the money spent on the disabled "employees" would be less than what the fines would have been. This practice is commonly called 挂靠/guakao—literally "to attach oneself to and rely on"—suggesting the tie of dependency that the disabled person develops with the company.[6]

My fieldwork shows that among all disabled groups, individuals with psychiatric disabilities are typically considered the least desirable choice for guakao, because companies often fear that they might appear at the workplace and make a fuss. Nevertheless, the meager benefits that guakao can provide are crucial to people with psychiatric disabilities and their families. Therefore, many caregivers have gone to great lengths to beg friends or street-level bureaucrats to introduce them to interested businesses. They hope that in so doing, their loved ones could become "workers" and enjoy paternalistic care (guan) from the "work units" as they themselves had in the past.

Through these vocal appeals and complicit actions, caregivers are striving for what I call a "paternalistic citizenship." They ask the state to recognize and compensate for their everyday work with patients, and they demand that the state assume paternalistic responsibilities for patients and themselves. Note that the meanings of this "paternalism" are manifold, and they can be observed in the different ways people invoke the term guan. First, caregivers demand that the state recognize their contributions to biopolitical paternalism—that is, the intimate management (guan) of people diagnosed with SMIs and deemed to be threats to the social order. Second, following the Confucian imagination of the state as a family writ large, caregivers ask the state to be a proper parent and care for (guan) all its offspring, particularly the most vulnerable—that is, people with SMIs and their family members. Third, clinging to the socialist ideology of state paternalism, caregivers urge the state to be responsible for (guan) them as former socialist workers and for those patients who can still claim a worker identity. In their everyday lives, particularly in collective discussions and actions, caregivers may strategically mobilize any or all of these paternalistic imaginaries, seeking to create intimate ties with the state and to break public/private boundaries.

In their attempts to claim paternalism citizenship, caregivers seek dependency on the very state they identify as the source of their suffering. Is that an effective strategy? If the state is hypocritical and prone to forgetting its paternal promises, can caregivers really take its words seriously? Indeed, my fieldwork shows some limits in these citizenship claims. Firstly, we have seen that in the Chinese context, the idea of paternalism is scalable, because its descriptive/prescriptive scope is able to contract or expand from the family to the state. Yet as anthropologists Summerson Carr and Michael Lempert (2016) remind us, scale-making projects are "institutionalizing projects, in which a particular way of being and seeing is socially enforced" (9). Caregivers may indeed scale up paternalism to the state to demand its support for patients and themselves, but state agents tend to use their discursive and institutional power to scale down paternalism and nail the responsibility on to the family. In the opening vignette, after Nan suggested that Qin ask the street-level bureaucrats to look after her husband, Qin said that it would be to no avail, because the bureaucrats would throw the ball back to her and emphasize her responsibility to *guan*, as a family member. For many caregivers I interviewed, this response is not a figment of their imagination but a reality they often face.

Moreover, as caregivers try to build paternalistic ties with government agencies or companies, they come to think of themselves and their loved ones as vulnerable beings who can only quietly maneuver or supplicate for the powerful party's benefits and mercy but cannot stand up to demand their rights. In December 2013, Aunt Gu from NAPMIF took me to the municipal Disabled Persons' Federation to discuss welfare issues concerning people with various disabilities. There, a few participants from other disability groups complained about the meager wages they had received from their *guakao* companies. A federation leader responded that the companies' practice was illegal. He asked workers to defend their right to a minimum wage and promised to provide them with legal aid. Aunt Gu anxiously chimed in: "It's not that people with psychiatric disabilities and us caregivers don't want to defend our rights. But we're afraid that if we do, the work units will immediately let us [people with psychiatric disabilities] go. After all, they are scared of us already. If that happens, we can't even hold onto the little benefits for which we've fought so hard. As individuals, we are very vulnerable."

In this meeting, Aunt Gu also raised the issue of social security and health insurance for people with psychiatric disabilities. To my surprise, she did not demand full government coverage for them. "I've surveyed all the family caregivers I know. 80% of us said that with some subsidies from the government, we are willing to pay the rest of the premium. You know, we are not trying to shirk our responsibility." She spoke so cautiously and made such a modest request, as if any slightly bolder move would irritate the government officials, giving them a reason to drop the issue once and for all. Later at BeWell, I witnessed similar caution when caregivers negotiated policy demands with state agents or imagined themselves to do so.

Scholars have suggested that the idea of socialist state paternalism not only requires that the state provide for its people but also requires people to reflect on what they have contributed to the state and to regard the state's difficulties as their own (Cho 2013). In our case, this spirit of self-criticism conjoins with the neoliberal discourse of self-responsibility to temper caregivers' political demands and collective action. Moreover, in Nanhua and across China, both advocacy associations like NAPMIF and service agencies like BeWell are sponsored and at least partially funded by local governments. Their caregivers, especially the leaders among them, understand that they must walk a fine line between pushing the government in their desired direction and assuming a collaborative or even submissive stance to maintain government endorsement. If, as Elizabeth Perry (2008) has argued, Chinese notions of rights and citizenship have always been characterized by collective membership in a polity that guarantees life and livelihood, then we should pay attention to how these notions are historically and institutionally contingent, binding specific expectations of the state with demands of its citizens.

Finally, in presenting people diagnosed with SMIs as vulnerable, caregivers often come to see them as incapable of independent living and decision-making, which contradicts their self-understandings and aspirations. For example, to address the problem of "the old nurturing the disabled" and to plan for after their own deaths, many caregivers have been asking local governments to build nursing homes and provide long-term residential care for patients. People diagnosed with SMIs typically frown on this idea, because they see themselves as capable of self-care (perhaps with some support) and want to live freely in the community. It is hard for them to be heard, because the government-sanctioned advocacy channels are dominated by agents of paternalism. For example, NAPMIF consists of family caregivers and mental health professionals, many of whom refuse to admit anyone diagnosed with mental illness as one of its members. "We [family caregivers] have to make decisions (做主/zuozhu) for patients," one of NAPMIF's core members said to me. "I don't want to sound rude, but you know, mentally ill patients have no brains."

As caregivers strategically highlight patients' violent potential to have their intimate labor of *guan* recognized, some of them have come to see their loved ones in this light. For instance, at BeWell, several caregivers vocally refused to include any patients in their entertainment activities, for fear of patients' volatility. Regardless of their own perspective, this advocacy strategy may backfire. Since 2016, various cities in China have responded to caregivers' requests and started subsidizing them for patient management work. These subsidies are higher than the existing care subsidies. Interestingly, for patients deemed to have a higher risk of violence, the management subsidies their caregivers receive far exceed those for caregivers of lower-risk patients (six thousand *yuan*/year vs. two thousand *yuan*/year in Nanhua in 2017), if caregivers in the former category are willing to send patients to a period of inpatient treatment. This arrangement is supposed to motivate caregivers to better manage high-risk patients and help them access medical resources. Some caregivers have complained to me that this policy is unfair, however: by tying money to patients' risk, it awards people who do poorly in patient management rather than those who do well. Some patients and even mental health professionals also worry that caregivers who want the money might fabricate signs of risk and have their loved ones hospitalized. If this policy response signals the state's increased willingness to act paternalistically, then these worries show that only the risk of violence and its management, not their needs or vulnerability, can bring people into the purview of this paternalism.

Creativity and Constraints on the State's Margins

In this chapter, we have traced how caregiving is constituted as a form of marginality in contemporary China. As anthropologists Veena Das and Deborah Pool (2004) suggest, life on the margins reflects and shapes "the political, regulatory, and disciplinary practices that constitute . . . 'the state'" (3), and instead of assuming passivity, we should look for "creativity of margins" in "how alternative forms of economic and political action are instituted" (19). In our case, we see that by asking people to fend for themselves and their family members, neoliberal social policies have denied vulnerabilities and needs for dependency amid mental illnesses. Such denials have trapped patients and caregivers in poverty, precarity, and everyday defeats. These experiences, along with their traumatic memories as former socialist workers, reveal to caregivers the state's hypocrisy—that is, the way it rhetorically invokes but practically abandons the promises of paternalistic care it has made to its people. These understandings allow them to righteously engage in complicit practices in search of welfare, health care, and leisure resources. Moreover, caregivers often refuse professionals' attempts to turn them into individual feeling subjects and to summon, discipline, and depoliticize their intimate labor. Instead, they co-construct narratives of suffering together, trace its source to sociopolitical injustice, and recruit others' help for change.

These common experiences of suffering and practices of creativity have formed a sociality among family caregivers. Instead of being based solely on biological knowledge and identification, this sociality intertwines understandings of patienthood and kinship with cultural-historical discourses of belonging and entitlement. Moreover, it allows family caregivers to traverse the public/private boundaries and make claims on state and market agents for themselves and patients alike. I have called such historically situated, relationally-oriented politics and practices "paternalistic citizenship" and have teased out its multiple discursive dimensions: seeking the state's recognition of familial labor in biopolitical paternalism, asking for the parent state to care for its vulnerable children, and demanding that the socialist state provide for its past and present workers. This paternalistic citizenship has allowed caregivers to successfully register certain requests for recognition and redistribution, but this also has its limits. The scalability of paternalism means that state agents can use their discursive and institutional power to pin paternalistic responsibilities on families. As dependents and even supplicants of state paternalism, caregivers have come to experience themselves as vulnerable to state (and corporate) power and have learned to temper their political demands with a spirit of self-responsibility. Finally, because biopolitical paternalism sees patients as vulnerable, incapable, and potentially violent, caregivers' advocacy along these lines may further stigmatize patients, subject them to institutional constraints, and reinforce the family as a site of not just risk management but also risk production.

The various dimensions of paternalistic citizenship can be, and have been, registered in the polysemous concept of *guan*. As theorists in advanced liberal contexts are concerned with how to politicize the often-privatized notion of care, the simultaneously intimate and political connotations of *guan* have allowed Chinese family caregivers to negotiate with the state in mutually intelligible ways. In particular, invocations around the historically mediated polysemy of *guan* have allowed caregivers to engage in complicit practices or stipulate explicit demands, and they have also enabled the state to both perform and deny responsibilities. In the Confucian cosmology of kinship/kingship, however, the state—or previously, the emperor—establishes superiority not only by claiming to be a father who rules (*guan*) its people but also, and more importantly, as a filial son who serves them (Zito 1997). I suspect that this idea of the filial state underlies caregivers' criticism of bureaucratic institutions that manage people instead of serving them. At any rate, when paternalism is registered solely in terms of *guan*, when it is overdetermined by conditions such as the withdrawal of the welfare state and the rise of population control, and when people are reduced to supplicants of the parent state, the potentials of paternalistic citizenship are circumscribed.

CONCLUSION

Resonance

In this book, I have traced the circulation, reconfiguration, and transformation of keywords such as *guan* to examine how mental health institutions, legal-administrative mechanisms, socioeconomic policies, and politico-cultural imaginations in contemporary China coalesce to shape the family's role in patient care and how people connect to their loved ones, live and plan for their lives, and demand social change. This journey has revealed a mode of governance called "biopolitical paternalism." It emerges as scientific and political discourses manufacture a kind of biological subject that must be managed and as the state claims to care for these subjects through management while displacing the actual responsibilities toward private structures, such as families. The labor of vulnerable caregivers supplements the work of biopolitical paternalism by fulfilling the management task while quietly challenging the assumptions of scientific mastery, state care, and intimate authority. The everyday workings of biopolitical paternalism then produce not only intimate injuries and ethical tension but also inequity across the population, because people's access to professional services is mediated by their families or other private relations, which in turn tend to be impoverished by all the responsibilities of care and management. Meanwhile, the simultaneous ideological legitimation and structural delegation of biopolitical paternalism opens new political potentials for people to make demands of the state.

While biopolitical paternalism has been identified in the mental health field, it has a wider existence and relevance in China. This is due to the lingering ideological attachments to Confucian and socialist paternalism, the widespread reconfiguration of the "people" into a biologized "population" that needs to be managed (Cho 2013; Dutton 2005), the devolution and uneven reconstruction of welfare and health care (Lee and Zhu 2006), and the rise of the security state (Lee and Zhang 2013). One can easily find resonances of biopolitical paternalism throughout the country. For example, the family planning policy has not only made married couples responsible for producing fewer—and now more—children but also children thought to be of better "quality" to save the nation-state from a "population crisis" (Anagnost 1995; Greenhalgh 2008). Child rearing is seen primarily as the responsibility of families, however, and it is difficult for struggling parents to secure public assistance. When a young child is severely disabled, the expensive medical bills, the added responsibility for care, and the child's perceived lack of "quality" cause some desperate parents to "abandon" them—that is, surreptitiously leave them to the public. These abandoned children are warehoused in state-run orphanages, which might divert them to foster families before hopefully having them adopted internationally. According to Erin Rafferty's (2023) ethnographic research, foster parents, most of whom are poor, elderly women, can form bonds with disabled children in ways that quietly resist the ableism, classism, and racism common in discourses of orphanage care and international adoption. Yet instead of recognizing such maternal care that enables disabled children to thrive, policymakers and experts are obsessed with preventing their birth by advocating for mandatory premarital and prenatal examinations (Ma 2014a). As such, both biological families and foster parents are configured as agents that realize the biopolitical paternalism of producing "good births" for the nation through their private and supplementary labor.

Under Xi Jinping's leadership, which started in 2012, the Chinese government has been more actively championing its "socialist superiority" over the West through programs that seek to protect biological lives and defend social stability. As such, biopolitical paternalism has intensified, with the state taking more direct action. For instance, in the mental health field, some cities have issued new policies to bring long-term hospitalization to individuals diagnosed with SMIS whose families cannot care for them, as an explicit attempt to "reduce risks to social control." During the COVID-19 pandemic, the Chinese state turned its entire citizenry, not just those with chronic illness or disability, into subjects of a heightened form of biopolitical paternalism. After the initial months of chaos, the state was able to use a "zero COVID" policy, which combined prolonged isolation of people remotely associated with positive cases, pervasive digital surveillance, and strict travel restrictions to keep cases at a low level. During the first two years, this policy largely allowed the state to claim a narrative of care for its people and one of success in controlling (管控/*guankong*) the pandemic vis-à-vis other countries (Sier 2021).

In reality, the state's containment apparatus struggled to keep up with the spread of the virus, especially after the highly transmissible Omicron variant arrived in China in late 2022. It had to extend in time and space to the point of disrupting the daily lives of nearly the entire populace. In some cases, the disruptions were manifested in bankruptcies, suicides, and untreated illnesses that led to traumatic deaths. It gradually dawned on people that the state saw them as virus carriers rather than human beings and that it cared more about its own image than their well-being (Sorace and Loubere 2022). The realization of the state's hypocrisy and indifference led to mass protests. In response to the protests, the failing economy, and rising case counts, the state abruptly ended all pandemic control measures in December 2022 without giving people access to effective mRNA vaccines, antiviral medications, or even basic fever medications. The upshot was rapid infections and a massive death toll, which were not acknowledged in official statistics (Woo and Cash 2022), as well as a general dismay with the state's lack of concern (不管/*buguan*). Whether under strict lockdown or its moratorium, people had to rely on their families, neighbors, and mutual aid groups for assistance (Ma, Bi, and Jiang, n.d.). Over the next few years, as China likely faces intensified geopolitical tension and continued economic stagnation, it will be worth tracking how the state reconfigures its role vis-à-vis biological life and the security of the body politic, as well as what horizons of social mobilization might open as people become disillusioned with both biopolitical paternalism and its absence.

Resemblance

In many countries, paternalism in the forms of guardianship and substitute decision-making by families exists and has historically been endorsed by law. For a few examples, starting from the eighteenth century, families in Japan could seek local authorities' permission to confine members deemed mad or otherwise incapacitated at home. In 1900, a law required each person with mental illness to be assigned a custodian who assumed all legal responsibilities on their behalf. These practices were to ensure the smooth functioning and continuation of the patriarchal household. In the late 1910s, psychiatric hospitals rose to prominence for confining people with mental illness, but families continued to hold the authority of initiating such confinement (Kim 2022). In nineteenth-century England, families sought court adjudication of lunacy to control property transactions by the seemingly weak-minded (Suzuki 2001). In the first half of the twentieth century, women deemed mentally ill in the United States could be committed to mental hospitals just because they had embarrassed their husbands or could not do housework (Metzl 2010). Recently, the world was shocked to learn of American pop singer Britney Spears' quest to end the conservatorship that had allowed her father to control her financial affairs and health care through claims of her mental illness (Harris et al. 2022). This reveals how persistent, pervasive, and potentially damaging practices of familial paternalism are. At any rate, although they seem to be private decisions, these practices are shaped by social norms, such as what makes a competent patriarch, a good wife, or a rational economic agent, and they also contribute to maintaining certain forms of social order.

Entangled with familial paternalism are institutional attempts to discipline people, often in the name of care. In Western Europe and North America, poorhouses were established as early as the seventeenth century to contain all kinds of social derelicts. In the eighteenth century, specialized institutions such as the psychiatric asylum emerged to rehabilitate particular kinds of subjects. Scientific knowledge played an increasingly important role in constructing these subjects, and the growing state power was willing to support the expansion of institutionalization. Since the mid-twentieth century, civil rights, deinstitutionalization, antipsychiatry, and other social movements have contributed to the waning of psychiatric hospitals and other total institutions. The receding welfare state has failed to provide sufficient community support for people freed from these spaces, however. Instead, it has worked with the ascending carceral state to produce a fragmented institutional landscape—from homeless shelters and community treatment programs to jails and prisons—where marginalized individuals are cycled through and service is combined with surveillance, coercion, or containment (Hopper et al. 1997). In late 2022, New York City Mayor Eric Adams announced a plan for police and emergency medical workers to forcibly remove homeless people suspected of having SMIs from streets and subways and take them to psychiatric hospitals for evaluation, even when they had not harmed anyone (Rajkumar 2022), thereby jeopardizing the tenuous achievements of deinstitutionalization.

Given these cases' resemblance of the situation in China, the concept of biopolitical paternalism could be useful for analyzing these tendencies. First, it resonates with the emerging literature in critical disability studies about how different institutional forms interlock (Chapman, Carey, and Ben-Moshe 2014). It further sheds light on their common logic of risk management, which casts people with mental illness or other disabilities as sources of familial and social disorder.

Second, biopolitical paternalism urges us to explore how familial/interpersonal paternalism intersects with, or how families and other private agents are implicated in, institutional discipline. In the United States, Reuben Miller (2021) has found that with its tough-on-crime fervor, the Clinton administration passed legislation to evict households with members or guests who had committed any crime on public housing premises; as a result, many families have had to turn away loved ones with criminal records or risk facing homelessness together. Paul Brodwin (2012) has documented how community mental health work uses lowly frontline caseworkers to control individuals with SMIs and to police their welfare access based on treatment compliance, which conflicts with the caseworkers' intention to care. Biopolitical paternalism guides us to further examine the mechanisms in which people are involved to perform paternalistic regulations like these and even come to see them as desirable, as well as the entangled vulnerability and intimate traumas that people experience when pitted against each other as the agents and subjects of such regulations.

Third, biopolitical paternalism requires us to understand the state not just as a set of institutions and their power effects but also as an ideological construct in relation to the family and other entities (Sharma and Gupta 2009). China is not the only country with cultural discourses of the "family state" (Borovoy 2012) or socialist legacies of state or corporate paternalism (Shever 2013). In fact, when an actual welfare state is absent or on the decline, people often come to desire a benevolent paternalistic state on which they can depend (Aretxaga 2003; Street 2012). These ideological attachments can be mobilized to legitimate the state's vision of subject regulation, turning people into "patients of the state" (Auyero 2012). Meanwhile, neoliberal discourses construct the family as a private unit of love and care that is of public import and private entities in general as more efficient in achieving public tasks than the state. With this in mind, we should interrogate how the state deploys the flexibility of the public/private divide—and the scalability of paternalism—to relegate tasks of subject regulation to these entities, while also educating, monitoring, or even directly intervening in them as it sees fit.

Reckoning

On September 27, 2017, after fifteen years of hospitalization, Xu Wei was finally released. In July that year, the Forensic Science and Technology Research Institute, under the Ministry of Justice, issued a statement certifying Wei's "full capacity for civil conduct," which meant that he could make decisions for himself. Wei walked out of the hospital with his girlfriend Yuanchun.[1] (Her elder brother had refused to sign for her discharge, and Wei's lawyer had spent much time convincing her adult son to take on guardianship and agree to her release.) Other patients at the hospital reportedly saw them off with loud cheers (Chen 2017). Of course, the activists who had supported him were thrilled with this result, including its implication that people diagnosed with SMIs do not necessarily lack legal capacity. They were hesitant to claim this as a victory, however. After all, they argued that legal capacity should be inherent in every human being; the fact that it had been evaluated and granted by forensic psychiatrists only reinforced the tyranny of the medical authority. Meanwhile, a psychiatrist familiar with the matter told me that the local court had not ruled in favor of Wei because no local entities had been willing to *guan* or be responsible for any potential violence after his discharge; now, the announcement from an institution directly under the Central government let everyone off the hook. Without the ability to assert pressure like Wei's team, however, it would have been difficult for other cases to receive this high-level involvement. Indeed, as of this writing, Wei's case has been the only one in which an inpatient has been able to sue a psychiatric hospital in China for discharge and gain freedom (Chen 2023).[2]

In December 2017, I visited Wei and Yuanchun at their home—a clean, cozy one-bedroom apartment in a faraway corner of Shanghai. With Wei's retirement pension of less than two thousand *yuan* per month as the only income, they had to rely on the support of Yuanchun's brother for everything from rent to food, but Wei was hopeful about the future. He was planning to start a nonprofit organization with several activist friends and help other inpatients. For him, this help did not mean getting everyone out, but it meant assisting people in evaluating what would be good for them. He argued that this was because "some people don't have the ability or the support to live alone. For the phrase 'supported autonomous decision-making,'[3] the lawyers emphasize autonomy, but I think support is really the most important." I asked him what support meant to him, and he said money.

Unfortunately, life has not turned out as planned for Wei. Before long, Yuanchun's family saw her as unstable and hospitalized her again, depriving Wei of both love and financial support. Partly because of China's tightened political environment, the organization he had hoped to establish did not materialize. As his life got stuck, he started to feel as if he was being followed and harassed by secret agents. In December 2018, he called me, saying that he was in Northeast China looking for work while trying to hide from followers and figuring out what was happening. He also asked me how to discern real feelings from false ones. I grew concerned and suggested that he return to Shanghai, apply for low-income housing, and talk to a social worker or therapist, because those resources either did not exist or were not available to him, a nonresident, in the Northeast. He became impatient, repeated that he was not mentally ill, and then hung up. I have not heard from him since. His activist friends told me that they had also suggested he see a psychiatrist and get on medication, which he refused. Because he developed a habit of going to the police station and incessantly complaining about his "harassers," they worried that he might be seen as a risk and forcibly hospitalized. If that happened, they said the media and the public would view it as proof that releasing patients had been a bad idea and that all patients should be locked up.

Rather than blaming Wei for his situation and its potential impact on patient rights advocacy, I tend to think it was the mental health system, including the advocacy work in opposition to but also situated within it, that was failing him. In our first meeting in 2014, Wei told me that he was fully aware of all the social expectations he carried, and I suspect that was why he had refused any psychiatric or professional help. After all, the normal/pathological divide undergirding the mental health legislative debates assumes that only the "normal" individual should be free and deserves dignity, whereas the pathological subject needs to be managed by whatever means. Operating under this assumption, Wei's struggle for freedom hinged on his insistence—to others and probably to himself—that he was completely "normal." Although the activists did try to destabilize this divide and claim legal capacity for everyone, it was more of an abstract idea than a concrete imagination of what it might take to live with vulnerability, alterity, *and* dignity (Kulick and Rydstrom 2015).

Support is what it takes, and Wei understood that. Unfortunately, the love for which he had longed had been taken from him, his chosen career had not panned out, and his welfare benefits were meager. The people and entities around him, such as his brothers and the residents' committee, wanted nothing to do with him. When I suggested that he seek help from a social worker or a therapist, I was not even sure how helpful the suggestion would be. After all, mental health social workers were few in number and mostly worked in psychiatric hospitals, sometimes just as office clerks; psychotherapy, though a growing service, was costly and mostly not covered by health insurance. Between the suffocating hospital and the shattered home, there seemed to be vast emptiness.

How, then, can we—as concerned scholars, activists, citizens, and people who may be living with or adjacent to disability—help people like Xu Wei disrupt the harm of biopolitical paternalism and co-construct a more caring society? Instead of accepting the division between the normal and the pathological, the manager and the managed, we should refuse the assumption that some people by nature require discipline. Even when we see ourselves as benefiting from the social "protection" that keeps risks at bay, we need to recognize how such mechanisms overgeneralize based on certain individual characteristics, sidestep interpersonal and structural processes that might have led to the apparently problematic behavior, and ignore alternative ways of being and healing, thereby inflicting damages on individuals, families, and other social relations. If China's pandemic policies are any guide, we should remind ourselves that we, like anyone else, could be subjected to these mechanisms.

Meanwhile, instead of equating rights with absolute autonomy, we should recognize human beings' inherent vulnerability, dependency, and need for support. Instead of treating any public intervention as a rights violation, we should press for policies and initiatives that provide resources for everyone—especially the more vulnerable individuals and their caregivers—to live a dignified life and that promote a wider and more just distribution of care responsibilities across society (Kittay 1999; Nishida 2022). Oftentimes, a good guide for our advocacy is caregivers' and recipients' desire for state paternalism, manifested in their open demands and comments as well as their quiet actions to assert or create identities of entitlement. Given that some of their desires are tempered by the neoliberal ideology of self- and familial responsibility, we should help them make bolder claims on the state, obliging it unconditionally to every one of its proudly dependent citizens (Ferguson 2015).

Besides bolder claims, more diverse notions of subjectivity and well-being must also be asserted than what biomedical and biopolitical notions have delimited. For that, we should follow the lead of the maternal, supplementary work people do to make lives livable. This work includes the home experiments that provide people with company and material comfort, that allow alternative ways of being to exist or even flourish, and that support people to adopt roles and identities meaningful to them. This includes the practical wisdom with which caregivers engage with the trauma and otherworldly experience of their loved ones. It also includes the reciprocal care that people with disabilities or otherwise cast in recipient roles extend to their caregivers, such as their ability to hold the latter in the joy and memories of intimate relations. Note that instead of blanket acceptance of the biological, heteronormative families and the harm they may impose, we should be mindful of alternative relations people build and families they choose, such as the ties between Uncle Huan and Sister Duo, Xu Wei and Yuanchun, the friendships that unite multiple caregivers and recipients in leisure activities, and the mutual aid groups that people form amid SMI, the pandemic, or other challenges. Of course, much of this supplemental work of healing and relationship building is messy and at times troubling, because it exists under the terms of biopolitical management and economic impoverishment. Instead of dismissing it, we need to look closely and empathically for what really matters to people in need, to listen to how they distinguish *guan* that nourishes from *guan* that suffocates and *buguan* that abandons. The answers to these questions, then, are what policies and services should enable and uplift from the supplementary labor of care.

Notes

1 Nanhua is a pseudonym, as are the names of most persons and organizations that I study. In China, psychiatric hospitals and other mental health agencies are few and far between, making them easily identifiable. To protect my interlocutors from potential sociopolitical repercussions, I anonymize not only their names, but also the organizations and places where they were located. When necessary, I also change any identifying details or present several persons/organizations/places as one. The only exceptions to the rule of anonymity apply to policymakers, leading psychiatrists, and human rights activists who have spoken publicly about psychiatry and the law.

2 In this case, the pseudonyms Xu Wei and Xu Xing were not made up by me, but widely used by the attorneys, activists, and journalists.

3 Xu Wei said he had merely scratched his father's face, whereas his brothers said he had broken his father's nose (Chen 2016b).

4 Around this time, some psychiatrists in China also started adopting a psychoanalytic lens in their work, to critique and intervene in what they saw as pathogenic dynamics in Chinese families. However, this trend was short-lived and did not pick back up until the 1980s. For a more detailed discussion of this development, see Ma (2014b).

5 Anthropologists have long argued that the ways people name, experience, express, and cope with distress differ across societies and are shaped by cultural systems of meaning (Benedict 1934; Kleinman 1991). Meanwhile, historians have shown that transformations of psychiatry and its understandings of madness/mental illness have been tied to society's changing notions of normality, reason, and morality (Porter 2002).

6 Building on these critiques, a Mad Pride movement has emerged to reclaim and champion people's lived experiences with madness/mental illness over professional knowledge, advocating for an anti-oppressive way of understanding and supporting them (Faulkner 2017; Lewis 2017; Menzies, LeFrançois, and Reaume 2013).

7 We follow historians and anthropologists' advice to not assume that the globalization of psychiatry is a uniform process but to heed how local actors selectively adapt, repurpose, and redefine ideas of psychiatry for their own agendas (Baum 2018; Kitanaka 2011; Zhang 2020).

8 The few critics that do consider the family tend to focus on its collaboration with psychiatric institutions (Goffman 1961) or the medicalization of family problems as individual disorders (Laing 1965).

9 For instance, disability studies scholars Stacy Clifford Simplican (2015) and Tom Shakespeare (2006) have criticized this tendency.

10 According to Michel Foucault, when population and security replaced sovereignty as the new focus of Euro-American governments in the eighteenth century, the family changed "from being a model to being a privileged instrument for the government" (Foucault 2009, 105; Donzelot 1979). Here, I draw inspiration from Foucault's discovery without assuming the same historical trajectory in China.

11 Similarly, Emmanuel Levinas argued that "the will to power is . . . the price which must sometimes be paid by the elevated thought of a civilization called to nourish persons and to lighten their sufferings" (Levinas 1988, 158–59).

12 Anthropologist Jianfeng Zhu and colleagues (2018) have also identified the importance and prevalence of *guan* in China's mental health services. They suggest that the culture of *guan* tends to "objectify and infantilize its subjects" (95) and turns families of people diagnosed with SMIs into agents of power. More needs to be said about the term's ideological purchase on families and the public as well as about its circulation, conceptualization, and contestation in different realms.

13 For example, in his review of paternalism in international humanitarianism and human rights practices, Barnett (2017) acknowledges that women, because of their perceived vulnerability, are often objects of paternalism. Nevertheless, he does not discuss the gendered dimension on the side of its agents. He also treats paternalism and maternalism as nearly synonymous, without examining how they connect or diverge.

14 Given the EJI's uniqueness, there is no point in anonymizing it.

1. CONSTRUCTING FAMILIES, CONTESTING PATERNALISMS

1 Because of the public nature of these cases and the legislative debates, I use either real names or common pseudonyms for people and organizations mentioned in this chapter instead of creating pseudonyms for them.

2 For a brief history of the kickbacks and price markup practices in drug sales in China, see Zhu (2011).

3 This phrase is inspired by Kim Hopper's phrase *the institutional circuit*, which refers to the "largely haphazard and uncoordinated transfers" of people with SMIs "across institutional domains" in the United States (Hopper et al. 1997, 664). Common across the American and Chinese circuits are the shortage of public health-care provisions and the fragmentation of patients' lives along the circuit.

4 For example, in 2010, administrators of a Shenzhen hospital asked a psychiatrist to secretly diagnose a nurse who had complained about wage disparities, and they then demoted her based on the diagnosis. The nurse sued the hospital and won the case (Liu and Wang 2011).

5 According to a 2009 media review, there had been over twenty reported cases of alleged wrongful hospitalization by families, employers, or local governments (Zhou 2009). The legal analysis report published by the EJI in 2010 reported ten such cases (Huang, Liu, and Liu 2010).

6 While many of the arguments raised by stakeholders in the legislative debates appeared in my interviews, I will quote their publicly available statements whenever available to give interested readers a taste of the public conversation at the time. This argument can be seen in Huang's Sina Weibo entry, May 21, 2011.

7 Huang's Sina Weibo entry, June 7, 2012.

8 Huang's Sina Weibo entry, December 19, 2012.

9 For instance, see Huang's Sina Weibo entry, July 21, 2011.

10 Huang's Sina Weibo entry, September 4, 2012.

11 Tang Hongyu, a forensic psychiatrist at the Peking University Institute of Mental Health and framer of the MHL, insisted that the principle of patient autonomy had existed in drafts of the law since the 1990s, and that the EJI did not facilitate its inclusion in the law (Wu 2016). Nevertheless, other leading psychiatrists such as Liu Xiehe (2012) and Michael Phillips and colleagues (2013) acknowledged the impact of the EJI's campaign and the controversies around "being mentally illed" on the law's emphasis on hospitalization procedures and the voluntary principle.

12 Huang's Sina Weibo entry, August 4, 2011.

13 For instance, Dr. Yu Xin, director of the Peking University Institute of Mental Health, commented along these lines on a global mental health panel in the 2015 conference of the Society for Psychological Anthropology held in Boston.

14 This phrase initially came from American psychiatrist Darold Treffert's (1973) criticism of the danger criterion of psychiatric commitment and its prioritization of patient autonomy. Not all Euro-American psychiatrists share this view. For example, Browning Hoffman (1977) argued: "Patients should not die with their rights on. But they should not live with their rights off, either" (68).

15 In the United States and some other advanced liberal countries, mental health legislation sometimes includes the terms *danger* and *risk* interchangeably when setting the threshold for involuntary hospitalization. Regardless of the term used, this phenomenon must be "immediate," "evidenced by a recent overt act, attempt or threat to do substantial harm to oneself or another," and "proved beyond a reasonable doubt" to justify "a massive curtailment of liberty" (Fitch and Swanson 2019, 4). As such, the criterion is strict and akin to what scholars of biopower have called "danger," the proof of which "can only be provided after the fact" (Castel 1991, 283). In contrast, risk, as these scholars view it, covers a wide range of factors that might influence, and are used to predict, future behavior.

16 Dr. Sun Dongdong made this comment at the aforementioned 2013 workshop.

2. HOSPITALIZATION, RISKS, AND FAMILIAL COMMITMENTS

1 For discussions on cultural experiences of femininity, blood, and madness, see Ma (2012).

2 Some male patients also claimed they had been suffering from unrequited love, neglect by partners, or other disorders in intimate relationships, but this was less common in my fieldwork. Perhaps it was easier for female patients to relate these experiences to me, a female researcher.

3 Fei Wu (2009) documented a similar quest for intimate justice in the case of suicide among rural women in Northern China.

4 In addition to *guan*, 治/*zhi* (the Chinese word for "treating" or "curing" disease) also has an underlying reference to administering, governing, and managing by bringing order to chaos.

5 Adam Hedgecoe (2001) calls this view of schizophrenia that prioritizes genetic factors the "diathesis-stressor model."

6 In fact, neuroscientists leading these neuroimaging studies of schizophrenia have argued that brain shrinkage is correlated with relapse duration, not the number of relapses (Andreasen et al. 2013). They have also debated about whether the use of antipsychotics might have caused brain shrinkage (Zipursky, Reilly, and Murray 2013), but the doctor at Benevolence did not mention this controversy.

3. KINSHIP AND ITS LIMITS AMID SERIOUS MENTAL ILLNESS

1 For a more thorough presentation and analysis of this story as it unfolded up to 2012, see Ma (2012).

2 The policy allowed couples with a disabled child to have a second child, but because SMIs are typically first diagnosed in early adulthood or late adolescence, it was often too late to have another child. This added to the feeling of tragedy for many parents.

3 Similarly, in the United States, some parents of children with intellectual or developmental disabilities have called for keeping institutionalization a choice, because otherwise they would have to shoulder the responsibility of care alone in the neoliberal economy (Ben-Moshe 2020).

4 不/*bu* means "no" or "not" in Chinese.

5 At BeWell, clients often addressed each other and were addressed by social workers in kinship terms to show familiarity, friendliness, and informality.

6 The term *sister* is typically used on young to middle-aged women whose marital status is ambiguous. It does not carry any religious implications.

7 For an extended discussion of the socialist legacy on psychological discourse in contemporary China, see Jie Yang (2015).

8 Similarly, anthropologists have discovered that in the United States, mothers are more likely to refrain from seeing their children from a (completely) pathological perspective and to develop alternative kinship imaginaries (Ginsburg and Rapp 2024; Landsman 2009).

4. BIOPOLITICAL PATERNALISM AND ITS MATERNAL SUPPLEMENTS IN COMMUNITY MENTAL HEALTH

A version of this chapter was published as "Biopolitical Paternalism and Its Maternal Supplements: Kinship Correlates of Community Mental Health Governance in China," *Cultural Anthropology* 35, no. 2 (May 2020): 290–316.

1 Among the media reports that feature home confinement and psychiatric unlocking, I chose to use the *New York Times* article because it concisely invokes several

key themes (the patient's violence, the caregiver's helplessness, and the doctor's heroic benevolence) and because the Peking University Mental Health Institute serves as the leading institution of the 686 Program.

2 Because these reports on home confinement—be they international or domestic— often end with psychiatrists going in and unlocking the patients or appealing for government-funded medical intervention, they were likely to have been orchestrated by the psychiatrists themselves or allied policymakers.

3 Anthropologist Mun Young Cho (2013) has discovered that instead of laid-off workers, people with disabilities have become the focus of the Chinese state's recent poverty relief efforts. According to her, this trend suggests the importance of concepts like population and biology in state governance.

4 For example, in a news feature published by the state's official news agency and clearly orchestrated by officials overseeing the community mental health program, the authors lamented the difficulty of calculating the number of domestic confinement cases but then claimed that over one million patients across China were under home confinement. The latter assertion was based on a rough estimate from Hebei Province, which in turn had been generalized from a small local sample within the province (Kong and Li 2013).

5 In Nanhua in 2013, an individual diagnosed with SMI could receive up to CNY 150 or USD 22 worth of medication per month, as well as a free basic physical checkup every three months.

6 In contrast, the phrase *regardless of occasion* in Levels 3 and 4 should be interpreted as "at an inappropriate occasion," often meaning outside the home.

7 The 关/*guan* in *guansuo* is a different Chinese character than the 管/*guan* discussed throughout the book.

8 The idea of the edge comes from Paul Brodwin and Livia Velpry's (2014) argument that no matter how passé or minor it may seem, institutional constraint still constitutes psychiatry's "rough edge of practice" (524).

9 My analysis of Dr. Gao's action in front of Uncle Long's house was inspired by Elana Buch's (2015) study of home care in Chicago, where she urged us to observe "doorway moments and boundary practices" for how people enact, reinscribe, or transform individual subject positions and broader social distinctions (45).

5. DETERMINING RISKS AND RESPONSIBILITIES UNDER THE MENTAL HEALTH LAW

1 The MHL is ambiguous on who can decide to discharge patients committed because of risks to others. It only states that doctors should regularly assess those patients' situations, and when they are fit for discharge, the doctors should notify their family members (National People's Congress 2012).

2 Anthropologist Carol Greenhouse (1986) has argued that paying too much attention to court cases will risk prioritizing rules over the sociocultural contexts in which rules operate. Instead, examining everyday practices related to legal processes can illuminate these contexts and the "power that the law generates in social systems" (32). While the emphasis on everyday practices is useful, this distinction

is problematic, for court cases also bring sociocultural contexts to bear. Hence my decision to explore both.

3 Note that this is different from the provision on involuntary hospitalization for treatment which, regardless of the agent, could only be implemented when risk is present. Nevertheless, in this and many other cases, because of family caregivers' needs for assistance, the determination of risk is at stake in both procedures, and people rarely distinguish between them.

4 In countries where psychiatric advance directives are common, a treating physician decides when a patient lacks decision-making capacity, and their advance directive must be followed. In fact, the advance directives are seen as tools that facilitate communication and collaboration between patients, caregivers, and professionals (SAMHSA 2019). It is unclear whether Dr. Jin was aware of these practices or whether he thought Huang would reject them.

5 In the United States, some of these situations are included in the criterion of "grave disability"—"an inability to provide for basic personal needs for food, clothing, or shelter"—qualifying a patient for involuntary hospitalization in most states. In a few states, grave disability falls under the definition of "danger to self" (Fitch and Swanson 2019, 9–10), but I have found no jurisdictions where perversion of the will—behavior contradicting what is commonly expected—is seen as a manifestation of grave disability.

6 Yang Shao and Bin Xie (2013), two leading psychiatrists involved in drafting national and local mental health legislation, also acknowledge that loosening the risk criteria "could intensify the public perception of individuals with mental disorders as 'dangerous,' and, thus, exacerbate the stigma and discrimination of persons with mental disorder" (384).

7 For example, Feng Jiang et al. (2018) examined case records of patients involuntarily admitted under the MHL from thirty-two psychiatric hospitals in twenty-nine provinces. They narrowly defined *risk* as referring only to "an attack on others/themselves or endangering public security or impulsive aggression" and found that only 45.3 percent of those patients had such risks when admitted. Through interviews with psychiatrists, Bo Chen (2023) has found that some now read any "abnormal" thought or action as dangerous. Ruiping Fan and Mingxu Wang (2015) point out that psychiatrists from several hospitals have come to ask caregivers to induce patients to engage in harmful behavior to qualify them for involuntary commitment.

8 Similarly, Luo et al. (2014) report that as of May 1, 2013, 1,033 of the 1,170 inpatients in a psychiatric hospital in Guangzhou had been there for over a year, and 64.6 percent of those long-term cases were because their caregivers had refused to let them out.

9 I cannot find any published paper with systematic comparisons to demonstrate this point. Still, it makes sense from the government's perspective because, unlike community mental health services, hospitalization does not cover every patient, and its costs are at least partly shouldered by families.

10 In particular, Huang suspected that the court's adjudication committee had been surreptitiously working on Xu Wei's case. An internal mechanism of a Chinese

court, this committee is composed of key members of the court and a representative from the corresponding level of the People's Congress. Its job is to review any case deemed complicated or of major social or legal consequence and to advise the presiding judge. Legal scholars have argued that it is through this committee that the will of the party-state infiltrates the supposedly independent legal process (He 2012).

11 See Story 2 in the Introduction for Xu Wei's comment.

6. SUFFERING, SOCIALITY, AND CITIZENSHIP AMONG FAMILY CAREGIVERS

A version of this chapter was published as "Affect, Sociality, and the Construction of Paternalistic Citizenship among Family Caregivers in China," *HAU: Journal of Ethnographic Theory* 11, no. 3 (February 2021): 958–71.

1 Scholars define this as households in which individuals over sixty years old (the mandated retirement age for most people) carry the sole/major responsibility of providing for people with disabilities with their own retirement pensions. In Shanghai, researchers found that as of 2012, there were 4,857 persons with disabilities who fell into this category, with the majority being persons with intellectual or mental disabilities (Shanghai Disabled Persons' Employment Service Center and School of Social Development at East China Normal University 2014). At BeWell, another team of researchers found that among the hundred or so families that had regularly participated in the center's activities in 2015, forty-six had familial arrangements which could be described as "the old nurturing the disabled" (reference not cited to maintain the site's anonymity).

2 Journalistic reports indicate that in 1985, the state coined the slogan, "It's good to have only one child; the state will care for you as you grow old" (只生一个好, 政府来养老/ *Zhi sheng yige hao, zhengfu lai yanglao*). In 1995, the promise was weakened to "It's good to have only one child; the state will help you as you grow old" (只生一个好, 政府帮养老/*Zhi sheng yige hao, zhengfu bang yanglao*). Recently, the slogan has become: "It's good to postpone retirement and provide for yourself as you grow old" (推迟退休好, 自己来养老/*Tuichi tuixiu hao, ziji lai yanglao*) (Chen and Xia 2013).

3 Uncle Huan claimed that in the early 1980s, while most workers received monthly salaries of only thirty to forty *yuan*, their original salaries should have been two hundred *yuan*; that is, the state had deducted more than one hundred fifty *yuan* for social security purposes. However, Mark Frazier (2005, 311) has pointed out that in typical SOEs, only 3 percent of the wage bill was set aside by unions in work units for benefits.

4 In contrast, the villagers in Central China that Steinmüller studied were embarrassed about their secretive practices, because they were attached to a discourse of scientific modernity and saw themselves as falling behind.

5 The clubhouse was shuttered in 2013 because of a funding shortage, and the sheltered workshop stopped giving trainees subsidies in 2019.

6 See R. Yang (2015) for an activist's account of the history of "quota scheme employment," especially its associated fines which support the Disabled Person

Employment Security Fund. See Xia and Zhang (2015) for an empirical study of the structural conditions for *guakao*, especially the complicity between companies, residents' committees, and people with disabilities.

1 Yuanchun, like Xu Wei, is a pseudonym used by the press.
2 In 2014, a psychiatric hospital in Liaoning sued the guardian (an adult son) of a patient for failing to bring him home when he had clinically recovered from bipolar disorder. The court ruled in favor of the hospital (Chen 2016a). Regardless, this case received no media coverage, and as of this writing, there have been no other cases of a hospital pursuing freedom for a patient.
3 The term is typically translated into "supported decision-making" in English, but its Chinese translation (支持性自主决策/*zhichixing zizhu juece*) includes the word *autonomous*.

References

Achtenberg, Hannah. 1983. "Mental Health Care in China." *Journal of Psychiatric Treatment and Evaluation* 5, no. 4: 371–75.

Adams, Vincanne, Michelle Murphy, and Adele E. Clarke. 2009. "Anticipation: Technoscience, Life, Affect, Temporality." *Subjectivity* 28, no. 1 (September): 246–65. https://doi.org/10.1057/sub.2009.18.

Agamben, Giorgio. 1998. *Homo Sacer: Sovereign Power and Bare Life.* Translated by Daniel Heller-Roazen. Palo Alto, CA: Stanford University Press.

Ahmed, Sara. 2014. *The Cultural Politics of Emotion.* London: Routledge.

Anagnost, Ann. 1995. "A Surfeit of Bodies: Population and the Rationality of the State in Post-Mao China." In *Conceiving the New World Order: The Global Politics of Reproduction*, edited by Faye Ginsburg and Rayna Rapp, 22–41. Berkeley: University of California Press.

Andreasen, Nancy C., Dawei Liu, Steven Ziebell, Anvi Vora, and Beng-Choon Ho. 2013. "Relapse Duration, Treatment Intensity, and Brain Tissue Loss in Schizophrenia: A Prospective Longitudinal MRI Study." *American Journal of Psychiatry* 170, no. 6 (June): 609–15. https://doi.org/10.1176/appi.ajp.2013.12050674.

Andreasen, Nancy C., Peg Nopoulos, Vincent Magnotta, Ronald Pierson, Steven Ziebell, and Beng-Choon Ho. 2011. "Progressive Brain Change in Schizophrenia: A Prospective Longitudinal Study of First-Episode Schizophrenia." *Biological Psychiatry* 70, no. 7 (October): 672–79. https://doi.org/10.1016/j.biopsych.2011.05.017.

Anonymous. 2009. "Bie rang fengkuang zai yan: Zou Yijun an He Jinrong an" [Don't let madness happen again: The cases of Zou Yijun and He Jinrong]. *Guangdong Wujian Shuofa* [Guangdong noontime legal report]. Accessed September 19, 2020.

Anonymous. 2010. "Hubei shangfang 'jingshen bingren' chuyuan zishu jingli, bei qiangpo chiyao" [Petitioning "psychiatric patient" in Hubei narrates his experience of being forced to take medication after discharge]. *Xinmin Net*, April 17, 2010. https://news.hsw.cn/system/2010/04/17/050488004.shtml.

Appelbaum, Paul S. 1994. *Almost a Revolution: Mental Health Law and the Limits of Change.* New York: Oxford University Press.

Aretxaga, Begoña. 2003. "Maddening States." *Annual Review of Anthropology* 32, no. 1 (October): 393–410. https://doi.org/10.1146/annurev.anthro.32.061002.093341.

Aulino, Felicity. 2016. "Rituals of Care for the Elderly in Northern Thailand: Merit, Morality, and the Everyday of Long-Term Care." *American Ethnologist* 43, no. 1 (February): 91–102. https://doi.org/10.1111/amet.12265.

Auyero, Javier. 2012. *Patients of the State: The Politics of Waiting in Argentina.* Durham, NC: Duke University Press.

Barlow, Tani. 1993. "Colonialism's Career in Postwar China Studies." *positions* 1, no. 1 (February): 224–67. https://doi.org/10.1215/10679847-1-1-224.

Barnett, Michael. 2017. "Introduction: International Paternalism: Framing the Debate." In *Paternalism beyond Borders*, edited by Michael Barnett, 1–44. Cambridge: Cambridge University Press.

Baum, Emily. 2018. *The Invention of Madness: State, Society, and the Insane in Modern China*. Chicago: University of Chicago Press.

Benedict, Ruth. 1934. "Anthropology and the Abnormal." In *An Anthropologist at Work; Writings of Ruth Benedict*, edited by Margaret Mead, 262–83. New York: Avon Books.

Ben-Moshe, Liat. 2020. *Decarcerating Disability: Deinstitutionalization and Prison Abolition*. Minneapolis: University of Minnesota Press.

Berlant, Lauren. 1999. "The Subject of True Feeling: Pain, Privacy, and Politics." In *Cultural Pluralism, Identity Politics, and the Law*, edited by Austin Sarat and Thomas Kearns, 49–83. Ann Arbor, MI: University of Michigan Press.

Biehl, João. 2005. *Vita: Life in a Zone of Social Abandonment*. Berkeley: University of California Press.

Biehl, João. 2010. "Human Pharmakon: Symptoms, Technologies, Subjectivities." In *A Reader in Medical Anthropology: Theoretical Trajectories, Emergent Realities*, edited by Byron J. Good, Michael M. J. Fischer, Sarah S. Willen, and Mary-Jo DelVecchio Good, 213–31. Hoboken, NJ: Wiley-Blackwell.

Blommaert, Jan. 2007. "Sociolinguistic Scales." *Intercultural Pragmatics* 4, no. 1 (March): 1–19. https://doi.org/10.1515/IP.2007.001.

Blumenthal, David, and William Hsiao. 2005. "Privatization and Its Discontents: The Evolving Chinese Health Care System." *New England Journal of Medicine* 353, no. 11 (September): 1165–70. https://doi.org/10.1056/nejmhpro51133.

Boris, Eileen, and Jennifer Klein. 2010. "Making Home Care: Law and Social Policy in the U.S. Welfare State." In *Intimate Labors: Cultures, Technologies, and the Politics of Care*, edited by Eileen Boris and Rachel Salazar Parreñas, 187–203. Palo Alto, CA: Stanford University Press.

Borovoy, Amy. 2012. "Doi Takeo and the Rehabilitation of Particularism in Postwar Japan." *Journal of Japanese Studies* 38, no. 2 (Summer): 263–95. https://doi.org/10.1353/jjs.2012.0056.

Bray, David. 2006. "Building 'Community': New Strategies of Governance in Urban China." *Economy and Society* 35, no. 4 (February): 530–49. https://doi.org/10.1080/03085140600960799.

Brodwin, Paul. 2012. *Everyday Ethics: Voices from the Front Line of Community Psychiatry*. Berkeley: University of California Press.

Brodwin, Paul, and Livia Velpry. 2014. "The Practice of Constraint in Psychiatry: Emergent Forms of Care and Control." *Culture, Medicine, and Psychiatry* 38, no. 4 (September): 524–26. https://doi.org/10.1007/s11013-014-9402-y.

Buch, Elana D. 2015. "Postponing Passage: Doorways, Distinctions, and the Thresholds of Personhood among Older Chicagoans." *Ethos* 43, no. 1 (March): 40–58. https://doi.org/10.1111%2Fetho.12071.

Buchanan, Allen. 1978. "Medical Paternalism." *Philosophy and Public Affairs* 7, no. 4 (Summer): 370–90.

Cao, Chengping. 2013. "Muqin shou han tielong, hanlei guan er 11 nian" [Mother with tears made an iron cage and locked her son inside for 11 years]. *Xinxi Ribao* [Information daily], May 27, 2013. http://edu.people.com.cn/n/2013/0527/c1053-21630106.html.

Carr, E. Summerson. 2010. *Scripting Addiction: The Politics of Therapeutic Talk and American Sobriety*. Princeton, NJ: Princeton University Press.

Carr, E. Summerson, and Michael Lempert. 2016. "Introduction: Pragmatics of Scale." In *Scale: Discourse and Dimensions of Social Life*, edited by E. Summerson Carr and Michael Lempert, 1–24. Berkeley: University of California Press.

Castel, Robert. 1991. "From Dangerousness to Risk." In *The Foucault Effect: Studies in Governmentality*, edited by Graham Burchell, Colin Gordon, and Peter Miller, 281–98. London: Harvester Wheatsheaf.

Chao, Ruth K. 1994. "Beyond Parental Control and Authoritarian Parenting Style: Understanding Chinese Parenting through the Cultural Notion of Training." *Child Development* 65, no. 4 (August): 1111–19. https://doi.org/10.2307/1131308.

Chapman, Chris, Allison C. Carey, and Liat Ben-Moshe. 2014. "Reconsidering Confinement: Interlocking Locations and Logics of Incarceration." In *Disability Incarcerated: Imprisonment and Disability in the United States and Canada*, edited by Liat Ben-Moshe, Chris Chapman, and Allison C. Carey, 3–24. New York: Palgrave MacMillan.

Chen, Bo. 2016a. "(2014) Shangsuren Wang Moujia yu bei shangsuren Liaoningsheng Fuyuan Junren Kangning Yiyuan, Wang Mouyi yiliao fuwu hetong jiufen, ershen" [(2014) Dispute over medical service contract between appellant Wang A and appellees Liaoning Veterans Psychiatric Hospital, Wang B, second trial]. *Sifa Caipan zhong de Jingshen Weisheng Fa* [Mental Health Law in trials], June 8, 2016. https://medium.com/@mentalhealthlaw.

Chen, Bo. 2016b. "Xu vs. the Hospital and His Guardian—Involuntary Inpatient Treatment." *International Journal of Mental Health and Capacity Law*, no. 22: 134–43. https://doi.org/10.19164/ijmhcl.v2016i22.498.

Chen, Bo. 2023. *Mental Health Law in China: A Socio-Legal Analysis*. London: Routledge.

Chen, Dan. 2013. "[Chen Dan su Beijing Huilongguan Yiyuan rengequan jiufen an] Shenli jieguo ji yuangao yijian" [(Chen Dan v. Beijing Huilongguan Hospital dispute over personality rights) Trial results and the plaintiff's opinion]. *CrazyWorld—Feiyue Fengrenyuan de Boke* [Blog of CrazyWorld—One flew over the cuckoo's nest], December 2, 2013. http://blog.sina.com.cn/s/blog_a89909680101erws.html.

Chen, Shaoming. 2007. "Ren yu buren: Rujia dexing lunli de yige quanshi xiangdu" [To endure or not endure: An interpretive perspective from Confucian virtue ethics]. *Xueshu Yuekan* [*Academic Monthly*] 39, no. 1: 60–65.

Chen, Si, and Yan Xia. 2013. "Yanglaojin 'kongzhang' shui lai tian?" [Who is to fill the "empty pension account"?]. *Guoji Jinrong Bao* [International finance], November 26, 2013. http://finance.people.com.cn/n/2013/1126/c1004-23652043.html.

Chen, Yang. 2012. "'Zhongzheng,' 'weihai' douyou jingshen binghuan caineng ruyuan"
[Involuntary commitment is only for psychiatric patients who are "seriously ill" and
"dangerous"]. *Xinkuaibao* [News express], December 18, 2012, A09. https://news
.sina.cn/sa/2012-12-18/detail-ikmyaawa4508541.d.html.

Chen, Yiping. 2017. "Jingshen Weisheng Fa diyi an yuangao lijing wunian susong,
chenggong 'feiyue fengrenyuan'" [The plaintiff of the first case under Mental Health
Law successfully "flew over the cuckoo's nest" after five years of lawsuit]. *The Paper*,
September 29, 2017. https://www.thepaper.cn/newsDetail_forward_1811048.

Cheng, Yu. 2015. "'Jingshen Weisheng Fa diyi an' yuangao baisu: qicaoren Liu Xiehe: Ta
gao cuo le!" [Plaintiff of "the first case under Mental Health Law" lost; Liu Xiehe,
drafter of the law: he sued the wrong party!]. *West China City Daily*, April 15, 2015.
https://news.sina.com.cn/o/2015-04-15/061931718941.shtml.

Cho, Mun Young. 2010. "On the Edge between 'the People' and 'the Population': Ethnographic Research on the Minimum Livelihood Guarantee." *China Quarterly* 201
(March): 20–37. https://doi.org/10.1017/S0305741009991056.

Cho, Mun Young. 2013. *The Specter of "the People": Urban Poverty in Northeast China*.
Ithaca, NY: Cornell University Press.

Cohen, Lawrence. 2013. "Given over to Demand: Excorporation as Commitment."
Contemporary South Asia 21, no. 3 (September): 318–32. https://doi.org/10.1080
/09584935.2013.826630.

Connell, Robert W., and James W. Messerschmidt. 2005. "Hegemonic Masculinity:
Rethinking the Concept." *Gender and Society* 19, no. 6 (December): 829–59. https://
doi.org/10.1177/0891243205278639.

Cooper, David. 1971. *Psychiatry and Anti-psychiatry*. New York: Ballantine Books.

Das, Veena, and Renu Addlakha. 2001. "Disability and Domestic Citizenship: Voice,
Gender, and the Making of the Subject." *Public Culture* 13, no. 3 (Fall): 511–31.
https://doi.org/10.1215/08992363-13-3-511.

Das, Veena, and Deborah Poole. 2004. "State and Its Margins: Comparative Ethnog-
raphies." In *Anthropology in the Margins of the State*, edited by Veena Das and
Deborah Poole, 3–34. New Delhi: Oxford University Press.

Davis, Deborah. 1993. "Urban Households: Supplicants to a Socialist State." In *Chinese
Families in the Post-Mao Era*, edited by Deborah Davis and Stevan Harrell, 50–76.
Berkeley: University of California Press.

Davis, Elizabeth Anne. 2012. *Bad Souls: Madness and Responsibility in Modern Greece*.
Durham, NC: Duke University Press.

Dean, Mitchell. 1998. "Risk, Calculable and Incalculable." *Soziale Welt* 49: 25–42.

de la Luz Ibarra, María. 2010. "My Reward is Not Money: Deep Alliances and End-
of-Life Care among Mexicana Workers and Their Wards." In *Intimate Labors:
Cultures, Technologies, and the Politics of Care*, edited by Rachel Salazar Parreñas
and Eileen Boris, 187–203. Palo Alto, CA: Stanford University Press.

Derrida, Jacques. 1997. *Of Grammatology*. Translated by Gayatri Spivak. Baltimore:
Johns Hopkins University Press.

Diamant, Neil. 2005. "Hollow Glory: The Politics of Rights and Identity among PRC
Veterans in the 1950s and 1960s." In *Engaging the Law in China: State, Society,*

and *Possibilities for Justice*, edited by Neil Diamant, Stanley Lubman, and Kevin J. O'Brien, 131–60. Palo Alto, CA: Stanford University Press.

Ding, Chunyan. 2014. "Involuntary Detention and Treatment of the Mentally Ill: China's 2012 Mental Health Law." *International Journal of Law and Psychiatry* 37, no. 6 (November–December): 581–88. https://doi.org/10.1016/j.ijlp.2014.02.032.

Donzelot, Jacques. 1979. *The Policing of Families*. New York: Pantheon Books.

Du, Xiao, and Yifan Feng. 2017. "Weishengfa zhuanjia jiedu 'shoushu qianzi' falv guiding" [Health law expert interprets legal stipulations on "surgery signatures"]. *Legal Daily*, September 8, 2017. https://www.sohu.com/a/190558632_260616.

Duckett, Jane. 2012. *The Chinese State's Retreat from Health: Policy and the Politics of Retrenchment*. London: Routledge.

Duckett, Jane, and Ana Inés Langer. 2013. "Populism versus Neoliberalism Diversity and Ideology in the Chinese Media's Narratives of Health Care Reform." *Modern China* 39, no. 6 (June): 653–80. https://doi.org/10.1177/0097700413492602.

Dumit, Joseph. 2012. *Drugs for Life: How Pharmaceutical Companies Define Our Health*. Durham, NC: Duke University Press.

Dutton, Michael. 2005. *Policing Chinese Politics: A History*. Durham, NC: Duke University Press.

Dworkin, Gerald. 1972. "Paternalism." *Monist* 56, no. 1 (January): 64–84. https://doi.org/10.5840/monist197256119.

Eichner, Maxine. 2017. "The Privatized American Family." *Notre Dame Law Review* 93, no. 1 (December): 213–66.

Evans, Harriet. 1996. *Women and Sexuality in China: Dominant Discourses of Female Sexuality and Gender since 1949*. New York: Continuum.

Evans, Harriet. 2017. "Patriarchal Investments: Expectations of Male Authority and Support in a Poor Beijing Neighborhood." In *Transforming Patriarchy: Chinese Families in the Twenty-First Century*, edited by Gonçalo Duro Dos Santos and Stevan Harrell, 182–99. Seattle: University of Washington Press.

Fan, Ruiping, and Mingxu Wang. 2015. "Taking the Role of the Family Seriously in Treating Chinese Psychiatric Patients: A Confucian Familist Review of China's First Mental Health Act." *Journal of Medicine and Philosophy* 40, no. 4 (August): 387–99. https://doi.org/10.1093/jmp/jhv014.

Faulkner, Alison. 2017. "Survivor Research and Mad Studies: The Role and Value of Experiential Knowledge in Mental Health Research." *Disability and Society* 32, no. 4 (March): 500–520. https://doi.org/10.1080/09687599.2017.1302320.

Fei, Xiaotong. 1962. *Peasant Life in China: A Field Study of Country Life in the Yangtze Valley*. London: Routledge and Kegan Paul.

Ferguson, James. 2015. *Give a Man a Fish: Reflections on the New Politics of Distribution*. Durham, NC: Duke University Press.

Fitch, W. Lawrence, and Jeffrey W. Swanson. 2019. *Civil Commitment and the Mental Health Care Continuum: Historical Trends and Principles for Law and Practice*. Rockville, MD: Substance Abuse and Mental Health Services Administration.

Fong, Vanessa L. 2004. *Only Hope: Coming of Age under China's One-Child Policy*. Palo Alto, CA: Stanford University Press.

Forman, Shepard. 1995. "Introduction." In *Diagnosing America: Anthropology and Public Engagement*, edited by Shepard Forman, 1–22. Ann Arbor, MI: University of Michigan Press.

Foucault, Michel. 1991. "Governmentality." In *The Foucault Effect: Studies in Governmentality*, edited by Graham Burchell, Colin Gordon, and Peter Miller, 87–104. London: Harvester Wheatsheaf.

Foucault, Michel. 2009. *Security, Territory, Population: Lectures at the Collège de France 1977–1978*. Translated by Graham Burchell. Edited by François Ewald and Alessandro Fontana. Vol. 4. London: Palgrave MacMillan.

Franklin, Sarah, and Susan McKinnon. 2001. "Relative Values: Reconfiguring Kinship Studies." In *Relative Values: Reconfiguring Kinship Studies*, edited by Susan McKinnon and Sarah Franklin, 1–25. Durham, NC: Duke University Press.

Fraser, Nancy. 1997. "From Redistribution to Recognition? Dilemmas of Justice in a 'Post-Socialist' Age." In *Justice Interruptus: Critical Reflections on the "Postsocialist" Condition*, edited by Nancy Fraser, 11–40. New York: Routledge.

Fraser, Nancy, and Linda Gordon. 1994. "A Genealogy of Dependency: Tracing a Keyword of the US Welfare State." *Signs* 19, no. 2 (Winter): 309–36. https://doi.org/10.1086/494886.

Frazier, Mark W. 2005. "What's in a Law? China's Pension Reform and Its Discontents." In *Engaging the Law in China*, edited by Neil Diamant, Stanley Lubman, and Kevin J. O'Brien, 108–30. Palo Alto, CA: Stanford University Press.

Friedman, Sara L. 2008. "The Intimacy of State Power: Marriage, Liberation, and Socialist Subjects in Southeastern China." *American Ethnologist* 32, no. 2 (January): 312–27. https://doi.org/10.1525/ae.2005.32.2.312.

Friedner, Michele, and Emily Cohen. 2015. "Inhabitable Worlds: Troubling Disability, Debility, and Ability Narratives." Somatosphere, April 20, 2015. https://somatosphere.net/2015/inhabitable-worlds-troubling-disability-debility-and-ability-narratives.html/.

Giddens, Anthony. 1999. "Risk and Responsibility." *Modern Law Review* 62, no. 1 (January): 1–10. https://doi.org/10.1111/1468-2230.00188.

Ginsburg, Faye, and Rayna Rapp. 2024. *Disability Worlds*. Durham, NC: Duke University Press.

Glosser, Susan L. 2003. *Chinese Visions of Family and State, 1915–1953*. Berkeley: University of California Press.

Goffman, Erving. 1961. *Asylums: Essays on the Social Situation of Mental Patients and Other Inmates*. Garden City, NY: Anchor Books.

Goffman, Erving. 1963. *Stigma: Notes on the Management of Spoiled Identity*. Englewood Cliffs, NJ: Prentice-Hall.

Gong, Jiakai, Shuhua Feng, and Quanyi Wang. 2005. "Jingshen weisheng gongzuo mianlin de xingshi he fazhan celue" [Situations and development strategies for mental health work]. *Beijing Medical Journal* 27, no. 8: 508–9.

Gong, Shaochun, and Hongming Chen. 2012. "Peng Baoquan: Meici kaiting zhiwei bijin zhenxiang" [Peng Baoquan: I repeatedly go to court only to seek truth]. *Xin Fazhi Bao* [New legal report], March 30, 2012.

Good, Byron J., and Mary-Jo DelVecchio Good. 2012. "Significance of the 686 Program for China and for Global Mental Health." *Shanghai Archives of Psychiatry* 24, no. 3 (June): 175–77. https://doi.org/10.3969%2Fj.issn.1002-0829.2012.03.008.

Good, Mary-Jo DelVecchio. 2001. "The Biotechnical Embrace." *Culture, Medicine and Psychiatry* 25, no. 4 (December): 395–410. https://doi.org/10.1023/a:1013097002487.

Government Administration Council of the Central People's Government, People's Republic of China. 1950. "Zhonghua Renmin Gongheguo Hunyin Fa" [The Marriage Law of the People's Republic of China]. March 3, 1950. http://www.npc.gov.cn /zgrdw/npc/lfzt/rlys/2014-10/24/content_1882723.htm.

Greenhalgh, Susan. 2008. *Just One Child: Science and Policy in Deng's China.* Berkeley: University of California Press.

Greenhalgh, Susan. 2020. "Governing through Science: The Anthropology of Science and Technology in Contemporary China." In *Can Science and Technology Save China?*, edited by Susan Greenhalgh and Li Zhang, 1–24. Ithaca, NY: Cornell University Press.

Greenhouse, Carol J. 1986. *Praying for Justice: Faith, Order, and Community in an American Town.* Ithaca, NY: Cornell University Press.

Gruijters, Rob J., and John Ermisch. 2019. "Patrilocal, Matrilocal, or Neolocal? Intergenerational Proximity of Married Couples in China." *Journal of Marriage and Family* 81, no. 3 (June): 549–66. https://doi.org/10.1111/jomf.12538.

Guan, Lili, Jin Liu, Xia Min Wu, Dafang Chen, Xun Wang, Ning Ma, Yan Wang, Byron Good, Hong Ma, and Xin Yu. 2015. "Unlocking Patients with Mental Disorders Who Were in Restraints at Home: A National Follow-Up Study of China's New Public Mental Health Initiatives." *PLoS One* 10, no. 4 (April): e0121425. https://doi .org/10.1371%2Fjournal.pone.0121425.

Hacking, Ian. 2000. *The Social Construction of What.* Cambridge, MA: Harvard University Press.

Haraway, Donna. 1991. *Simians, Cyborgs, and Women: The Reinvention of Nature.* New York: Routledge.

Harders, Ann-Cathrin. 2012. "Ius Vitae Necisque." In *The Encyclopedia of Ancient History*, edited by Roger S. Bagnall, Kai Brodersen, Craige Brian Champion, Andrew Erskine, and Sabine R. Huebner, 3559–60. Malden, MA: Wiley-Blackwell.

Harrell, Stevan, and Gonçalo Duro Dos Santos. 2017. "Introduction." In *Transforming Patriarchy: Chinese Families in the Twenty-First Century*, edited by Gonçalo Duro Dos Santos and Stevan Harrell, 3–38. Seattle: University of Washington Press.

Harris, Lesley M., Sara M. Williams, Eva X. Nyerges, and Rebecka Bloomer. 2022. "Teaching Note—Beyond #Freebritney: Teaching Social Workers about Surrogate Decision Making through the Spears Case." *Journal of Social Work Education* 60, no. 1 (October): 140–54. https://doi.org/10.1080/10437797.2022.2119065.

Harvey, David. 2007. *A Brief History of Neoliberalism.* New York: Oxford University Press.

He, Li. 2009. "Jintian ni 'bei xx' le ma—'bei shidai' yujing xia de ganga yu wunai" [Have you been . . . today? Embarrassment and helplessness in the "era of passivity"]. *Xinhua Net*, July 31, 2009.

He, Xin. 2012. "Black Hole of Responsibility: The Adjudication Committee's Role in a Chinese Court." *Law and Society Review* 46, no. 4 (December): 681–712. https://doi .org/10.1111/j.1540-5893.2012.00514.x.

Heberer, Thomas, and Christian Göbel. 2011. *The Politics of Community Building in Urban China*. New York: Routledge.

Hedgecoe, Adam. 2001. "Schizophrenia and the Narrative of Enlightened Gene- ticization." *Social Studies of Science* 31, no. 6 (December): 875–911. https://doi.org /10.1177/030631201031006004.

Hoffman, Browning. 1977. "Living with Your Rights Off." *Bulletin of the American Acad- emy of Psychiatry and the Law* 5, no. 1: 68–74.

Hofmann, J. Allen. 1913. "A Report of the Patients Discharged from the John G. Kerr Hospital for Insane during 1912," *China Medical Journal* 27, no. 6 (November): 369–79.

Hopper, Kim, John Jost, Terri Hay, Susan Welber, and Gary Haugland. 1997. "Homeless- ness, Severe Mental Illness, and the Institutional Circuit." *Psychiatric Services* 48, no. 5 (May): 659–65. https://doi.org/10.1176/ps.48.5.659.

Hou, Ying. 2010. "'Bei shidai' de yuyanxue jiedu" [Linguistic interpretation of the "era of passivity"]. *Xiandai Yuwen* [*Modern Chinese*], no. 2: 136–39.

Hsu, Francis L. K. 1971. *Under the Ancestor's Shadow*. Palo Alto, CA: Stanford Univer- sity Press.

Huang, Hsuan-Ying. 2015. "From Psychotherapy to Psycho-Boom: A Historical Over- view of Psychotherapy in China." *Psychoanalysis and Psychotherapy in China* 1, no. 1 (June): 1–30. https://doi.org/10.4324/9780429478772-1.

Huang, Xin. 2014. "In the Shadow of Suku (Speaking-Bitterness): Master Scripts and Women's Life Stories." *Frontiers of History in China* 9, no. 4 (December): 584–610. https://doi.org/10.3868/s020-003-014-0039-6.

Huang, Xuetao, Xiaohu Liu, and Jiajia Liu. 2010. "Zhongguo Jingshenbing Shouzhi Zhidu Falv Fenxi Baogao" [The involuntary commitment system in China: A critical analysis]. Shenzhen: Equity and Justice Initiative, October 10, 2010. http:// rpdstudies.cn/d/file/p/2019/03-03/5ab5bd842599770c4c08b96339ecd4e1.pdf.

Jain, Sarah Lochlann. 2007. "Living in Prognosis: Toward an Elegiac Politics." *Represen- tations* 98, no. 1 (Spring): 77–92. https://doi.org/10.1525/rep.2007.98.1.77.

Jia, Fujun. 2010. "Jiankang quan yeshi renquan" [The right to health is also a human right]. Chinese Psychiatrist Association, November 9, 2010.

Jiang, Feng, Huixuan Zhou, Jeffrey J. Rakofsky, Linlin Hu, Tingfang Liu, Huanzhong Liu, Yuanli Liu, and Yi-lang Tang. 2018. "The Implementation of China's Mental Health Law-Defined Risk Criteria for Involuntary Admission: A National Cross- Sectional Study of Involuntarily Hospitalized Patients." *Frontiers in Psychiatry* 9 (November): 560. https://doi.org/10.3389/fpsyt.2018.00560.

Jinan Shenkang Hospital. n.d. "Shenkang jiesuo jiuzhu jishi—Liu Yaxin baituo tiesuo shengya" [Shenkang's record of unlocking and rescuing Liu Yaxin]. Accessed March 23, 2017. http://www.jnskyy.com/mtbd/shyf/14522.html.

Kao, John J. 1979. *Three Millennia of Chinese Psychiatry*. New York: Institute for Ad- vanced Research in Asian Science and Medicine.

Kerr, John G. 1898. "The 'Refuge for the Insane', Canton." *China Medical Missionary Journal* 12, no. 4: 177–78.

Kim, Eunjung. 2017. *Curative Violence: Rehabilitating Disability, Gender, and Sexuality in Modern Korea*. Durham, NC: Duke University Press.

Kim, H. Yumi. 2022. *Madness in the Family: Women, Care, and Illness in Japan*. New York: Oxford University Press.

Kipnis, Andrew. 2006. "Suzhi: A Keyword Approach." *China Quarterly* 186 (July): 295–313. https://doi.org/10.1017/S0305741006000166.

Kitanaka, Junko. 2011. *Depression in Japan: Psychiatric Cures for a Society in Distress*. Princeton, NJ: Princeton University Press.

Kittay, Eva Feder. 1999. *Love's Labor: Essays on Women, Equality, and Dependency*. New York: Routledge.

Kleinman, Arthur. 1991. *Rethinking Psychiatry: From Cultural Category to Personal Experience*. New York: Simon and Schuster.

Kleinman, Arthur. 2009a. "Caregiving: The Odyssey of Becoming More Human." *Lancet* 373, no. 9660 (January): 292–93. https://doi.org/10.1016/s0140-6736(09)60087-8.

Kleinman, Arthur. 2009b. "Global Mental Health: A Failure of Humanity." *Lancet* 374, no. 9690 (August): 603–4. https://doi.org/10.1016/S0140-6736(09)61510-5.

Klinke, Ian. 2013. "Chronopolitics: A Conceptual Matrix." *Progress in Human Geography* 37, no. 5 (February): 673–90. https://doi.org/10.1177/0309132512472094.

Kohrman, Matthew. 2003. "Why Am I Not Disabled? Making State Subjects, Making Statistics in Post-Mao China." *Medical Anthropology Quarterly* 17, no. 1 (March): 5–24. https://doi.org/10.1525/maq.2003.17.1.5.

Kong, Pu, and Tianyu Li. 2013. "Long zhong ren" [Men in cages]. *Beijing Xinwen* [*Beijing News*], July 11, 2013. http://www.bjnews.com.cn/feature/2013/07/11/272800.html.

Kowalski, Julia. 2016. "Ordering Dependence: Care, Disorder, and Kinship Ideology in Antiviolence Counseling in North India." *American Ethnologist* 43, no. 1 (February): 63–75. https://doi.org/10.1111/amet.12263.

Kuan, Teresa. 2015. *Love's Uncertainty: The Politics and Ethics of Childrearing in Contemporary China*. Berkeley: University of California Press.

Kulick, Don, and Jens Rydstrom. 2015. *Loneliness and Its Opposite: Sex, Disability, and the Ethics of Engagement*. Durham, NC: Duke University Press.

LaFraniere, Sharon. 2010. "Life in Shadows for Mentally Ill in China." *New York Times*, November 10, 2010, A1.

Laing, R. D. 1965. *The Divided Self: An Existential Study in Sanity and Madness*. New York: Penguin Books.

Landsman, Gail H. 2009. *Reconstructing Motherhood and Disability in the Age of "Perfect" Babies*. New York: Routledge.

Large, Matthew M., Christopher James Ryan, Olav B. Nielssen, and R. A. Hayes. 2008. "The Danger of Dangerousness: Why We Must Remove the Dangerousness Criterion from Our Mental Health Acts." *Journal of Medical Ethics* 34, no. 12 (December): 877–81. https://doi.org/10.1136/jme.2008.025098.

Lazarus-Black, Mindie, and Susan F. Hirsch, eds. 1994. *Contested States: Law, Hegemony, and Resistance*. New York: Routledge.

Lee, Ching Kwan, and Yonghong Zhang. 2013. "The Power of Instability: Unraveling the Microfoundations of Bargained Authoritarianism in China." *American Journal of Sociology* 118, no. 6 (May): 1475–508. https://doi.org/10.1086/670802.

Lee, Haiyan. 2007. *Revolution of the Heart: A Genealogy of Love in China, 1900–1950.* Palo Alto, CA: Stanford University Press.

Lee, James, and Ya-peng Zhu. 2006. "Urban Governance, Neoliberalism and Housing Reform in China." *Pacific Review* 19, no. 1 (November): 39–61. https://doi.org/10.1080/09512740500417657.

Lee, Sing. 2001. "From Diversity to Unity: The Classification of Mental Disorders in 21st-Century China." *Psychiatric Clinics of North America* 24, no. 3 (September): 421–31. https://doi.org/10.1016/s0193-953x(05)70238-0.

Levinas, Emmanuel. 1988. "Useless Suffering." In *The Provocation of Levinas: Rethinking the Other,* edited by Robert Bernasconi and David Wood, 156–67. New York: Routledge.

Lewis, Bradley. 2017. "A Mad Fight: Psychiatry and Disability Activism." In *The Disability Studies Reader,* edited by Lennard Davis, 102–18. New York: Routledge.

Li, Gang. 2013. "Teshu jiating: Feiyue jingshenbingyuan" [A special family: One flew over the cuckoo's nest]. *Beijing Youth News,* June 3, 2013.

Li, Ke-Qing, Xiu-li Sun, Yong Zhang, Guang Shi, and Arnulf Kolstad. 2012. "Zhongguo jingshen weisheng fuwu jiqi zhengce: Dui 1949–2009 nian de huigu ji weilai 10 nian de zhanwang" [Mental health services in China: A review of delivery and policy issues in 1949–2009]. *Zhongguo Xinli Weisheng Zazhi* [*Chinese Mental Health Journal*] 26, no. 5: 321–26.

Lin, Tsung-Yi, and Mei-Chen Lin. 1980. "Love, Denial and Rejection: Responses of Chinese Families to Mental Illnesses." In *Normal and Abnormal Behavior in Chinese Culture,* edited by Arthur Kleinman and Tsung-Yi Lin, 387–402. Boston: Kluwer.

Lin, Zhuyun, and Zhiying Ma. 2023. "When Psychiatry Encounters Local Knowledge of Madness: Ethnographic Observations in a Chinese Psychiatric Hospital." *SSM—Mental Health* 4 (September): 100266. https://doi.org/10.1016/j.ssmmh.2023.100266.

Liu, Chunlin, and Ying Wang. 2011. "Bei danwei xuanbu wei 'jingshenbing,' Shenzhen yi hushi daying guansi" [Announced by work unit to be mentally ill, a Shenzhen nurse won the case]. *South China Metropolis,* May 9, 2011.

Liu, Xiehe. 2012. "A Long Overdue Pleasure." *Shanghai Archives of Psychiatry* 24, no. 6 (December): 359. https://doi.org/10.3969%2Fj.issn.1002-0829.2012.06.010.

Lord, Janet E., and Michael Ashley Stein. 2013. "Contingent Participation and Coercive Care: Feminist and Communitarian Theories of Disability and Legal Capacity." In *Coercive Care: Rights, Law and Policy,* edited by Bernadette McSherry and Ian Freckleton, 31–48. New York: Routledge.

Lovell, Anne M., and Lorna A. Rhodes. 2014. "Psychiatry with Teeth: Notes on Coercion and Control in France and the United States." *Culture, Medicine, and Psychiatry* 38, no. 4 (November): 618–22. https://doi.org/10.1007/s11013-014-9420-9.

Luhrmann, Tanya M. 2011. *Of Two Minds: An Anthropologist Looks at American Psychiatry.* New York: Vintage.

Luo, Zhixin, Xiangjiao Liao, Zhimei Xie, Erlang Hong, Fengkun Chang, Liqun Li, Shuai Gao, et al. 2014. "Jingshen Weisheng Fa shishi hou jingshen bingren changqi zhuyuan yuanyin diaocha" [Causes of long-term hospitalization after the implementation of the Mental Health Law.] *China Journal of Health Psychology* 22, no. 12: 1769–71.

Ma, Hong, Jin Liu, Yanling He, Bin Xie, Yifeng Xu, Wei Hao, Hongyu Tang, Mingyuan Zhang, and Xin Yu. 2011. "Zhongguo jingshen weisheng fuwu moshi gaige de zhong-yao fangxiang: 686 moshi" [An important pathway of mental health service reform in China: Introduction of 686 Program]. *Chinese Mental Health Journal* 25, no. 10: 725–28.

Ma, Zhiying. 2012. "Psychiatric Subjectivity and Cultural Resistance: Experience and Explanations of Schizophrenia in Contemporary China." In *Chinese Modernity and the Individual Psyche*, edited by Andrew Kipnis, 203–28. New York: Palgrave MacMillan.

Ma, Zhiying. 2014a. "Guanyu 'qiying dao,' cong canzhang he zhaoliao jiaodu shuo jiju" [Observation on "safety islands" from the perspectives of disability and care]. *Youren Zazhi* [Youren magazine] 2, no. 2: 22.

Ma, Zhiying. 2014b. "An 'Iron Cage' of Civilization? Missionary Psychiatry and the Making of a 'Chinese Family' at the Turn of the Century." In *Psychiatry and Chinese History*, edited by Howard Chiang, 91–110. London: Pickering and Chatto.

Ma, Zhiying. 2022. "Invitation from Disability." *Fieldsights*, September 6, 2022. https://culanth.org/fieldsights/invitation-from-disability.

Ma, Zhiying, Yaochu Bi, and Naiyu Jiang. "Pandemic, Paternalism, and the Possibili-ties of Citizenship in China: A Netnography." *American Ethnologist*. Revise and resubmit.

Maddux, James E., and Barbara A. Winstead, eds. 2019. *Psychopathology: Foundations for a Contemporary Understanding*. New York: Routledge.

Martin, Patricia Yancy. 2004. "Gender as Social Institution." *Social Forces* 82, no. 4 (June): 1249–73. https://doi.org/10.1353/sof.2004.0081.

Mason, Katherine. 2016. *Infectious Change: Reinventing Chinese Public Health after an Epidemic*. Palo Alto, CA: Stanford University Press.

Mattingly, Cheryl. 2014. *Moral Laboratories: Family Peril and the Struggle for a Good Life*. Berkeley: University of California Press.

McKinnon, Susan, and Fenella Cannell. 2013. "The Difference Kinship Makes." In *Vital Relations: Modernity and the Persistent Life of Kinship*, edited by Susan McKinnon and Fenella Cannell, 3–38. Santa Fe, NM: School for Advanced Research Press.

Menzies, Robert, Brenda A. LeFrançois, and Geoffrey Reaume. 2013. "Introducing Mad Studies." In *Mad Matters: A Critical Reader in Canadian Mad Studies*, edited by Brenda A. LeFrançois, Robert Menzies, and Geoffrey Reaume, 1–22. Toronto: Canadian Scholars' Press.

Metzl, Jonathan. 2010. *The Protest Psychosis: How Schizophrenia Became a Black Dis-ease*. Boston: Beacon Press.

Metzl, Jonathan, and Anna Kirkland. 2010. "Against Health." In *Against Health: How Health Became the New Morality*, edited by Anna Kirkland and Jonathan Metzl, 1–11. New York University Press.

Miller, Reuben Jonathan. 2021. *Halfway Home: Race, Punishment, and the Afterlife of Mass Incarceration*. New York: Little, Brown and Company.

Ministry of Health, People's Republic of China. 2012. *Yanzhong Jingshen Zhang'ai Guanli Zhiliao Gongzuo Guifan* [Working rules for management and treatment of serious mental illnesses]. April 12, 2012. http://www.nhc.gov.cn/jkj/s5888/201204/16ebc49bfe504f979eb31070fc3ac5bf.shtml.

Mol, Annemarie. 2002. *The Body Multiple: Ontology in Medical Practice*. Durham, NC: Duke University Press.

Mol, Annemarie, Ingunn Moser, and Jeannette Pols. 2010. "Care: Putting Practice into Theory." In *Care in Practice: On Tinkering in Clinics, Homes and Farms*, edited by Annemarie Mol, Ingunn Moser, and Jeannette Pols, 7–26. Piscataway, NJ: Transcript Verlag.

Myers, Neely Laurenzo. 2015. *Recovery's Edge: An Ethnography of Mental Health Care and Moral Agency*. Nashville: Vanderbilt University Press.

Nader, Laura. 1969. *Law in Culture and Society*. Berkeley: University of California Press.

Nakamura, Karen. 2013. *A Disability of the Soul: An Ethnography of Schizophrenia and Mental Illness in Contemporary Japan*. Ithaca, NY: Cornell University Press.

National People's Congress, People's Republic of China. 1980. *Zhonghua Renmin Gongheguo Hunyin Fa* [The Marriage Law of the People's Republic of China]. September 10, 1980.

National People's Congress, People's Republic of China. 1986. *Zhonghua Renmin Gongheguo Minfa Tongze* [General Principles of the Civil Law of the People's Republic of China]. April 12, 1986.

National People's Congress, People's Republic of China. 1996. *Zhonghua Renmin Gongheguo Laonianren Quanyi Baozhang Fa* [Law of the People's Republic of China on Protection of the Rights and Interests of the Elderly]. August 29, 1996. http://www.npc.gov.cn/zgrdw/wxzl/gongbao/1996-08/29/content_1479994.htm.

National People's Congress, People's Republic of China. 2011. *Jingshen Weisheng Fa (Cao'an) Tiaowen ji Tiaowen Shuoming* [Mental Health Law (draft) and explanations]. October 29, 2011.

National People's Congress, People's Republic of China. 2012. *Zhonghua Renmin Gongheguo Jingshen Weisheng Fa* [Mental Health Law of the People's Republic of China]. Beijing: Law Press China.

New, Bill. 1999. "Paternalism and Public Policy." *Economics and Philosophy* 15, no. 1 (December): 63–83. https://doi.org/10.1017/s0266267100000359x.

Ng, Emily. 2009. "Heartache of the State, Enemy of the Self: Bipolar Disorder and Cultural Change in Urban China." *Culture, Medicine, and Psychiatry* 33, no. 3 (September): 421–50. https://psycnet.apa.org/doi/10.1007/s11013-009-9144-4.

Nguyen, Vinh-Kim. 2005. "Antiretroviral Globalism, Biopolitics, and Therapeutic Citizenship." In *Global Assemblages: Technology, Politics, and Ethics as Anthropological Problems*, edited by Aihwa Ong and Stephen Collier, 124–44. Malden, MA: Wiley-Blackwell.

Nishida, Akemi. 2022. *Just Care: Messy Entanglements of Disability, Dependency, and Desire*. Philadelphia: Temple University Press.

Nussbaum, Martha Craven. 2006. *Frontiers of Justice: Disability, Nationality, Species Membership*. Cambridge, MA: Harvard University Press.

Ong, Aihwa, and Li Zhang. 2008. "Introduction: Privatizing China, Powers of the Self, Socialism from Afar." In *Privatizing China: Socialism from Afar*, edited by Li Zhang and Aihwa Ong, 1–19. Ithaca, NY: Cornell University Press.

Pan, Zhongde, Bin Xie, and Zhanpei Zheng. 2003. "Woguo jingshen zhang'aizhe de ruyuan fangshi diaocha" [A survey on psychiatric hospital admission and related factors in China]. *Journal of Clinical Psychological Medicine* 13, no. 5: 270–74.

Pearson, Veronica. 1995. *Mental Health Care in China: State Policies, Professional Services and Family Responsibilities*. London: Gaskell.

Peking University Sixth Hospital. 2016. "Zhongyang buzhu difang yanzhong jingshen zhang'ai guanli zhiliao xiangmu" [Program for managing and treating serious mental illnesses, run by local governments and subsidized by the central government]. August 31, 2016. https://www.pkuh6.cn/Html/News/Articles/2486.html.

Peng, Man-Man, Zhiying Ma, and Mao-Sheng Ran. 2022. "Family Caregiving and Chronic Illness Management in Schizophrenia: Positive and Negative Aspects of Caregiving." *BMC Psychology* 10, no. 1 (March): 83. https://doi.org/10.1186%2Fs40359-022-00794-9.

Perry, Elizabeth J. 2008. "Chinese Conceptions of 'Rights': From Mencius to Mao—and Now." *Perspectives on Politics* 6, no. 1 (February): 37–50. https://doi.org/10.1017/S1537592708080055.

Petryna, Adriana. 2004. "Biological Citizenship: The Science and Politics of Chernobyl-Exposed Populations." *Osiris* 19, no. 1: 250–65. https://doi.org/10.1086/649405.

Phillips, Michael R. 1993. "Strategies Used by Chinese Families Coping with Schizophrenia." In *Chinese Families in the Post-Mao Era*, edited by Stevan Harrell and Deborah Davis, 277–306. Berkeley: University of California Press.

Phillips, Michael R. 1998. "The Transformation of China's Mental Health Services." *China Journal* 39 (January): 1–36. https://doi.org/10.2307/2667691.

Phillips, Michael R., Hanhui Chen, Kate Diesfeld, Bin Xie, Hui G. Cheng, Graham Mellsop, and Xiehe Liu. 2013. "China's New Mental Health Law: Reframing Involuntary Treatment." *American Journal of Psychiatry* 170, no. 6 (June): 588–91. https://doi.org/10.1176/appi.ajp.2013.12121559.

Pinto, Sarah. 2014. *Daughters of Parvati: Women and Madness in Contemporary India*. Philadelphia: University of Pennsylvania Press.

Porter, Roy. 2002. *Madness: A Brief History*. New York: Oxford University Press.

Povinelli, Elizabeth. 2006. *The Empire of Love: Toward a Theory of Intimacy, Genealogy, and Carnality*. Durham, NC: Duke University Press.

Rabinow, Paul. 1996. "Artificiality and Enlightenment." In *Essays on the Anthropology of Reason*, edited by Paul Rabinow, 91–111. Princeton, NJ: Princeton University Press.

Rafferty, Erin. 2023. *Families We Need: Disability, Abandonment, and Foster Care's Resistance in Contemporary China*. New Brunswick, NJ: Rutgers University Press.

Rajkumar, Shruti. 2022. "Advocates Fear the Impact of NYC's Involuntary Hospitalization Plan." *HuffPost*, December 13, 2022. https://www.huffpost.com/entry/nyc-homeless-plan-ugly-laws_n_63991195e4b0169d76dba769.

Rapp, Rayna, and Faye Ginsburg. 2011. "Reverberations: Disability and the New Kinship Imaginary." *Anthropological Quarterly* 84, no. 2 (Spring): 379–410. https://doi.org /10.1353/anq.2011.0030.

Read, Benjamin. 2012. *Roots of the State: Neighborhood Organization and Social Networks in Beijing and Taipei.* Palo Alto, CA: Stanford University Press.

Rembis, Michael. 2017. "Introduction." In *Disabling Domesticity*, edited by Michael Rembis, 1–23. New York: Palgrave MacMillan.

Reyes-Foster, Beatriz. 2018. *Psychiatric Encounters: Madness and Modernity in Yucatan, Mexico.* New Brunswick, NJ: Rutgers University Press.

Rosaldo, Renato. 1994. "Anthropology and 'the Field.'" Conference held at Stanford University and UC Santa Cruz, February 18–19.

Rose, Nikolas. 1996. "The Death of the Social? Re-figuring the Territory of Government." *Economy and Society* 25, no. 3 (July): 327–56. https://doi.org/10.1080 /03085149600000018.

Rose, Nikolas, and Peter Miller. 1992. "Political Power beyond the State: Problematics of Government." *British Journal of Sociology* 43, no. 2 (June): 173–205.

Rosenberg, Charles. 2007. *Our Present Complaint: American Medicine, Then and Now.* Baltimore: Johns Hopkins University Press.

Ross, Robert. 1920. "The Treatment of the Insane." *China Medical Journal* 34, no. 5: 580–81.

Ross, Robert. 1926. "Mental Hygiene." *China Medical Journal* 40, no. 1: 8–13.

Rubinstein, Ellen B. 2018. "Extraordinary Care for Extraordinary Conditions: Constructing Parental Care for Serious Mental Illness in Japan." *Culture, Medicine and Psychiatry* 42, no. 4 (December): 755–77. https://doi.org/10.1007/s11013-018-9595-6.

Ruddick, Sara. 1995. *Maternal Thinking: Toward a Politics of Peace.* Boston: Beacon Press.

Saari, Jon L. 1990. *Legacies of Childhood: Growing up Chinese in a Time of Crisis, 1890–1920.* Cambridge, MA: Harvard University Asia Center.

Sahlins, Marshall. 2011. "What Kinship is (Part One)." *Journal of the Royal Anthropological Institute* 17, no. 1 (March): 2–19. https://doi.org/10.1111/j.1467-9655.2010 .01666.x.

SAMHSA (Substance Abuse and Mental Health Services Administration). 2019. *A Practical Guide to Psychiatric Advance Directives.* Rockville, MD: Center for Mental Health Services.

Sarat, Austin, and Thomas Kearns. 1995. "Beyond the Great Divide: Forms of Legal Scholarship and Everyday Life." In *Law in Everyday Life*, edited by Austin Sarat and Thomas Kearns, 21–61. Ann Arbor: University of Michigan Press.

Scheper-Hughes, Nancy. 1993. *Death without Weeping: The Violence of Everyday Life in Brazil.* Berkeley: University of California Press.

Scott, Joan W. 1999. "Gender: A Useful Category of Historical Analysis." In *Gender and the Politics of History*, edited by Joan W. Scott, 28–50. New York: Columbia University Press.

Selden, Charles. 1909a. "II. Treatment of the Insane." *China Medical Journal* 23, no. 4: 221–32.

Selden, Charles. 1909b. "III. Treatment of the Insane." *China Medical Journal* 23, no. 6: 373–84.

Selden, Charles. 1910. "The Need of More Hospitals for Insane in China." *China Medical Journal* 24, no. 5: 325–30.

Shakespeare, Tom. 2006. *Disability Rights and Wrongs*. London: Routledge.

Shanghai Disabled Persons' Employment Service Center and School of Social Development at East China Normal University. 2014. "'Lao yang can' jiating xianzhuang ji sikao: Yi Shanghai Shi weili" [Family condition of disabled people cared for by the elderly in Shanghai and some further thoughts: Taking Shanghai as an example]. *Disability Research* 1: 13–18.

Shanghai Municipal People's Congress. 2001. "Shanghai Shi Jingshen Weisheng Tiaoli" [Mental Health Ordinance of the city of Shanghai]. December 28, 2001.

Shanghai No.1 Interm. People's Ct., People's Republic of China. 2015. Xu v. the Hospital and His Guardian—Involuntary Inpatient Treatment.

Shao, Yang, and Bin Xie. 2013. "Operationalizing the Involuntary Treatment Regulations of China's New Mental Health Law." *Shanghai Archives of Psychiatry* 25, no. 6 (December): 384–86. https://doi.org/10.3969/j.issn.1002-0829.2013.06.007.

Shao, Yang, Bin Xie, Mary-Jo Good, and Byron Good. 2010. "Current Legislation on Admission of Mentally Ill Patients in China." *International Journal of Law and Psychiatry* 33, no. 1 (January–February): 52–57. https://doi.org/10.1016/j.ijlp.2009.10.001.

Sharma, Aradhana, and Akhil Gupta. 2009. "Rethinking Theories of the State in an Age of Globalization." In *The Anthropology of the State: A Reader*, edited by Aradhana Sharma and Akhil Gupta, 1–41. New York: John Wiley and Sons.

Shever, Elana. 2013. "'I Am a Petroleum Product': Making Kinship Work on the Patagonian Frontier." In *Vital Relations: Modernity and the Persistent Life of Kinship*, edited by Susan McKinnon and Fenella Cannell, 85–108. Santa Fe, NM: School for Advanced Research Press.

Shorter, Edward. 1998. *A History of Psychiatry: From the Era of the Asylum to the Age of Prozac*. New York: John Wiley and Sons.

Sier, Willy. 2021. "The Politics of Care during COVID-19: The Visibility of Anti-virus Measures in Wuhan." *China Information* 35, no. 3 (July): 274–300. https://doi.org/10.1177/0920203X211032370.

Silverman, Chloe. 2011. *Understanding Autism: Parents, Doctors, and the History of a Disorder*. Princeton, NJ: Princeton University Press.

Simonis, Fabien. 2010. "Mad Acts, Mad Speech, and Mad People in Late Imperial Chinese Law and Medicine." PhD diss., Princeton University.

Simplican, Stacy Clifford. 2015. "Care, Disability, and Violence: Theorizing Complex Dependency in Eva Kittay and Judith Butler." *Hypatia* 30, no. 1 (November): 217–33. https://doi.org/10.1111/hypa.12130.

Solinger, Dorothy J. 2006. "The Creation of a New Underclass in China and Its Implications." *Environment and Urbanization* 18, no. 1 (April): 177–93. https://doi.org/10.1177/0956247806063972.

Song, Shaopeng. 2012. "Ziben zhuyi, shehui zhuyi he funv—Weishenme zhongguo xuyao chongjian Makesi zhuyi nvquan zhuyi pipan" [Capitalism, socialism, and women: Why China needs to rebuild Marxist feminist critiques]. *Open Times* 12: 98–112.

Sorace, Christian. 2018. "Extracting Affect: Televised Cadre Confessions in China." *Public Culture* 31, no. 1 (January): 145–71. https://doi.org/10.1215/08992363-7181871.

Sorace, Christian, and Nicholas Loubere. 2022. "Biopolitical Binaries (or How Not to Read the Chinese Protests)." *Made in China Journal,* December 2, 2022. https://madeinchinajournal.com/2022/12/02/biopolitical-binaries-or-how-not-to-read-the-chinese-protests/.

Soss, Joe, Richard C. Fording, and Sanford Schram. 2011. *Disciplining the Poor: Neoliberal Paternalism and the Persistent Power of Race.* Chicago: University of Chicago Press.

Speed, Ewen. 2006. "Patients, Consumers and Survivors: A Case Study of Mental Health Service User Discourses." *Social Science and Medicine* 62, no. 1 (January): 28–38. https://doi.org/10.1016/j.socscimed.2005.05.025.

Stacey, Judith. 1983. *Patriarchy and Socialist Revolution in China.* Berkeley: University of California Press.

Steinmüller, Hans. 2010. "Communities of Complicity: Notes on State Formation and Local Sociality in Rural China." *American Ethnologist* 37, no. 3 (July): 539–49. https://doi.org/10.1111/j.1548-1425.2010.01271.x.

Steinmüller, Hans. 2015. "'Father Mao' and the Country-Family: Mixed Feelings for Fathers, Officials, and Leaders in China." *Social Analysis* 59, no. 4 (December): 83–100. https://doi.org/10.3167/sa.2015.590406.

Stevenson, Lisa. 2014. *Life Beside Itself: Imagining Care in the Canadian Arctic.* Berkeley: University of California Press.

Stonington, Scott. 2020. *The Spirit Ambulance: Choreographing the End of Life in Thailand.* Berkeley: University of California Press.

Street, Alice. 2012. "Seen by the State: Bureaucracy, Visibility and Governmentality in a Papua New Guinean Hospital." *Australian Journal of Anthropology* 23, no. 1 (February): 1–21. https://doi.org/10.1111/j.1757-6547.2012.00164.x.

Suzuki, Akihito. 2001. "Enclosing and Disclosing Lunatics in the Family Walls: Domestic Psychiatric Regime and the Public Sphere in Early Nineteenth-Century England." In *Outside the Walls of the Asylum: The History of Care in the Community 1750–2000,* edited by Peter Bartlett and David Wright, 115–31. London: The Athlone Press.

Szasz, Thomas. 1964. *The Myth of Mental Illness: Foundations of a Theory of Personal Conduct.* New York: Harper and Row.

Tang, Hongyu. 2010. "Feiziyuan zhuyuan de juedaduoshu shi zhenzheng jingshenbing huanzhe" [The overwhelming majority of persons involuntarily hospitalized are real psychiatric patients]. Chinese Psychiatrist Association, November 9, 2010.

Taylor, Janelle S. 2008. "On Recognition, Caring, and Dementia." *Medical Anthropology Quarterly* 22, no. 4 (December): 313–35. https://doi.org/10.1111/j.1548-1387.2008.00036.x.

Tomba, Luigi. 2014. *The Government Next Door: Neighborhood Politics in Urban China.* Ithaca, NY: Cornell University Press.

Treffert, Darold. 1973. "Dying with Their Rights On." *American Journal of Psychiatry* 130, no. 9 (April): 1041. https://doi.org/10.1176/ajp.130.9.1041.

Tronto, Joan C. 1993. *Moral Boundaries: A Political Argument for an Ethic of Care.* London: Psychology Press.

Tsing, Anna. 2012. "On Scalability: The Living World is Not Amenable to Precision-Nested Scales." *Common Knowledge* 18, no. 3 (August): 505–24. https://doi.org/10.1215/0961754X-1630424.

United Nations General Assembly. 2007. *Convention on the Rights of Persons with Disabilities and Optional Protocol.* New York: United Nations.

Verdery, Katherine. 1996. *What Was Socialism, and What Comes Next?* Princeton, NJ: Princeton University Press.

Walder, Andrew G. 1988. *Communist Neo-Traditionalism: Work and Authority in Chinese Industry.* Berkeley: University of California Press.

Wang, Jing. 2009. "Sun Dongdong: Ba jingshen bingren songdao yiyuan shi zuida de baozhang" [Sun Dongdong: Hospitalizing the mentally ill is the greatest protection]. *China News Weekly,* March 18, 2009.

Wang, Mengqi. 2018. "'Rigid Demand': Economic Imagination and Practice in China's Urban Housing Market." *Urban Studies* 55, no. 7 (May): 1579–94. https://doi.org/10.1177/0042098017747511.

Wang, Peilian, and Xinling Li. 2012. "Beijing Huilongguan Yiyuan yuanzhang: 'Bei jingshenbing' butai rongyi" [Director of Beijing Huilongguan Hospital: It's not that simple to "be mentally illed"]. *China Youth Daily,* July 4, 2012. https://zqb.cyol.com/html/2012-07/04/nw.D110000zgqnb_20120704_4-03.htm.

Whyte, Martin King. 2005. "Continuity and Change in Urban Chinese Family Life." *China Journal* 53 (January): 9–33. https://doi.org/10.2307/20065990.

Williams, Raymond. 1985. *Keywords: A Vocabulary of Culture and Society.* New York: Oxford University Press.

Wolf, Margery. 1972. *Women and the Family in Rural Taiwan.* Palo Alto, CA: Stanford University Press.

Wolfe, Cary. 2008. "Introduction: Exposures." In *Philosophy and Animal Life,* edited by Stanley Cavell, Cora Diamond, John McDowell, Ian Hacking, and Cary Wolfe, 1–42. New York: Columbia University Press.

Woo, Ryan, and Joe Cash. 2022. "China COVID Deaths Accelerate to 9,000 a day—UK Research Firm Airfinity." *Reuters,* December 29, 2022. https://www.reuters.com/world/china/china-covid-deaths-accelerate-9000-day-uk-research-firm-airfinity-2022-12-29/.

Woods, Andrew. 1923. "A Memorandum to Chinese Medical Students on the Medicolegal Aspects of Insanity." *National Medical Journal of China* 9: 203–12.

World Health Organization. 2011a. *Mental Health Atlas 2011.* Geneva, Switzerland.

World Health Organization. 2011b. *Mental Health Atlas 2011—China.* Geneva, Switzerland.

Wu, David Y. H. 1996. "Parental Control: Psychocultural Interpretations of Chinese Patterns of Socialization." In *Growing up the Chinese Way: Chinese Child and Adolescent Development,* edited by Sing Lau, 1–28. Hong Kong: Chinese University Press.

Wu, Fei. 2009. *Suicide and Justice: A Chinese Perspective*. London: Routledge.

Wu, Harry Yi-Jui. 2016. "The Moral Career of 'Outmates': Towards a History of Manu-factured Mental Disorders in Post-socialist China." *Medical History* 60, no. 1 (January): 87–104. https://doi.org/10.1017/mdh.2015.70.

Wu, Zhiguo, and Bin Xie. 2011. "Jingshen zhang'ai feiziyuan yiliao de Zhongguo shijiao he tansuo" [The views and exploration on involuntary mental health care in China]. *Chinese Journal of Health Policy* 4, no. 9: 10–15.

Xi, Nan. 2013. "Bei jingshenbing de 72 xiaoshi" [72 hours of being mentally illed]. *Beijing Evening News*, November 6, 2013.

Xia, Changbao, and Jiangyue Zhang. 2015. "Canjiren zheng jiuye: Qiye, shequ juweihui, canjiren jian de xingwei luoji fenxi—yi X shequ weili" [Employment of disability certificates: Analyzing the behavioral logics of companies, residents' committees, and people with disabilities, with Community X as an example]. *Disability Research* 4: 30–36.

Xie, Bin, and Hong Ma. 2011a. "Jingshenbing feiziyuan yiliao zhende name kepa ma?" [Is involuntary psychiatric treatment really so horrifying?]. *Caixin*, June 20, 2011. https://china.caixin.com/m/2011-06-20/100271328.html.

Xie, Bin, and Hong Ma. 2011b. "Youguan Jingshen Weisheng Fa de liuge misi" [Six myths concerning the Mental Health Law]. *Tianma Xingkong 2006's Blog*, June 18, 2011. https://www.psychspace.com/psych/viewnews-4724.

Xie, Bin, Hongyu Tang, and Hong Ma. 2011. "Jingshen weisheng lifa de guoji shiye he Zhongguo xianshi: Laizi Zhongguo Yishi Xiehui Jingshenke Yishi Fenhui de guandian" [Gap between international routine and reality of China: Problems reflected in the legislation process of Chinese Mental Health Law]. *Chinese Mental Health Journal* 25, no. 10: 721–24.

Xishu. 2018. "Zhongguo ban Feiyue Fengrenyuan: Mimou shiqi nian de taowang" [One flew over the cuckoo's nest in China: An escape secretly planned over 17 years]. *Zhenshi Gushi Jihua* [Truman story], March 25, 2018. https://www.douban.com/note/662967607/.

Xu, Jing. 2017. *The Good Child: Moral Development in a Chinese Preschool*. Palo Alto, CA: Stanford University Press.

Yan, Yunxiang. 1997. "The Triumph of Conjugality: Structural Transformation of Family Relations in a Chinese Village." *Ethnology* 36, no. 3 (Summer): 191–212. https://doi.org/10.2307/3773985.

Yan, Yunxiang. 2016. "Intergenerational Intimacy and Descending Familism in Rural North China." *American Anthropologist* 118, no. 2 (April): 244–57. https://doi.org/10.1111/aman.12527.

Yan, Yunxiang. 2018. "Neo-Familism and the State in Contemporary China." *Urban Anthropology and Studies of Cultural Systems and World Economic Development* 47, no. 3–4 (Fall–Winter): 181–224. https://doi.org/10.2307/45172908.

Yanagisako, Sylvia Junko, and Jane Fishburne Collier. 1987. "Toward a Unified Analysis of Gender and Kinship." In *Gender and Kinship: Essays Toward a Unified Analysis*, edited by Jane Fishburne Collier and Sylvia Junko Yanagisako, 14–50. Palo Alto, CA: Stanford University Press.

Yang, Chengxin. 2012. "Jingshen Weisheng Fa zhong 'sifa chengxu' yu 'guojia fuquan' de zhongyaoxing" [The importance of "legal procedures" and "state paternalism" in the Mental Health Law]. *Yang Chengxin's Blog*, August 31, 2012. https://china.caixin.com /2012-10-16/100447760.html.

Yang, Jie. 2015. *Unknotting the Heart: Unemployment and Therapeutic Governance in China*. Ithaca, NY: Cornell University Press.

Yang, Renliang. 2015. "Canbaojin zhong you xin dongtai? Pandian naxie liangdian yu changdao" [Finally some new developments of the Disabled Person Employment Security Fund? An inventory of policy highlights and activism]. *Yang Renliang's Blog*, September 17, 2015.

Yngvesson, Barbara. 1988. "Making Law at the Doorway: The Clerk, the Court, and the Construction of Community in a New England Town." *Law and Society Review* 22, no. 3: 409–48. https://doi.org/10.2307/3053624.

Zelizer, Viviana A. 2005. *The Purchase of Intimacy*. Princeton, NJ: Princeton University Press.

Zhang, Baolin. 2017. "Duanping: Guangzhou Huang laotai shijian gei women de qishi" [Comments: Reflections on the Mrs. Huang incident in Guangzhou]. *Zhongguo Zhili Canjiren ji Qinyou Xiehui* [China Association of Persons with Intellectual Disability and their Relatives], November 1, 2017.

Zhang, Li. 2001. "Migration and Privatization of Space and Power in Late Socialist China." *American Ethnologist* 28, no. 1 (February): 179–205. https://doi.org/10.1525 /ae.2001.28.1.179.

Zhang, Li. 2012. *In Search of Paradise: Middle-Class Living in a Chinese Metropolis*. Ithaca, NY: Cornell University Press.

Zhang, Li. 2020. *Anxious China: Inner Revolution and Politics of Psychotherapy*. Berkeley: University of California Press.

Zhang, Ran. 2013a. "Jingshen Weisheng Fa xiayue shishi, jianhuren bu jie huanzhe chuyuan huo bei su" [Mental Health Law to be implemented next month; guardians who don't discharge patients may be sued]. *Jinghua Shibao* [*Jinghua Times*], April 18, 2013.

Zhang, Ran. 2013b. "Jingshen zhang'ai fangzhi duoge wenti daijie" [Many problems to be solved for the prevention and treatment of mental disorders]. *Beijing Times*, April 18, 2013.

Zhang, Yanhua. 2007. *Transforming Emotions with Chinese Medicine: An Ethnographic Account from Contemporary China*. Albany: State University of New York Press.

Zhao, Zhenhuan. 2008. *Jingshenke Linchuang Jineng Caozuo Shouce* [Manual of clinical techniques for psychiatrists]. Guangzhou, China: Jinan University Press.

Zhou, Hualei. 2009. "Nvzi yin 'jiating jiufen' bei qiangxing songjin jingshenbingyuan yinfa guanzhu" [Woman forcefully hospitalized because of "family conflict," drawing public attention]. *China News Weekly*, March 25, 2009. http://www.chinanews .com/jk/ysbb/news/2009/03-25/1617665.shtml.

Zhu, Hengpeng. 2011. "Yaopin ling chajia zhidu de houguo" [Consequences of the zero markup for drug sales rule]. *Caixin*, January 26, 2011. https://zhuhengpeng.blog .caixin.com/archives/4748.

Zhu, Jianfeng, Tianshu Pan, Hai Yu, and Dong Dong. 2018. "Guan (Care/Control): An Ethnographic Understanding of Care for People with Severe Mental Illness from Shanghai's Urban Communities." *Culture, Medicine and Psychiatry* 42, no. 1 (March): 92–111. https://doi.org/10.1007/s11013-017-9543-x.

Zhu, Xi. 2013. *Lunyu Jizhu* [Collected notes on the Analects]. Beijing: Zhongguo Shehui Chubanshe [China society publishing house].

Zhu, Yuanhong. 1992. "Pragmatic Feudalism: Narrative Analysis of Collective Memory, Using Post-1949 Mainland China as a Case." *Journal of Chinese Sociology* 16: 1–23.

Zipursky, Robert B., Thomas J. Reilly, and Robin M. Murray. 2013. "The Myth of Schizophrenia as a Progressive Brain Disease." *Schizophrenia Bulletin* 39, no. 6 (November): 1363–72. https://doi.org/10.1093%2Fschbul%2Fsbs135.

Zito, Angela. 1997. *Of Body and Brush: Grand Sacrifice as Text/Performance in Eighteenth-Century China*. Chicago: University of Chicago Press.

Index

to, 98–101; and home confinement problem, 101–7; home visits in, 96–103, 107, 120; methodology in research on, 23–24; risk management in, 27, 89–90, 95–98, 101, 104, 107–8; 686 Program in (*see* 686 Program)

compassion, 12, 83–84, 90; in covert medications, 98–101; as feminized and devalued, 105; in home confinement, 104–7; and unbearable burden of suffering, 104–7

compliance with medications, 17, 65, 72; in covert administration, 99, 108; family responsibility for, 53, 64–65, 66, 82; and relapse risk, 66, 73, 113–14; side effects affecting, 52, 64, 73

Confucianism, 5, 11, 156; compassion in, 105; family-state isomorphism in, 19, 41; filiality in, 8, 10, 19, 154; kinship in, 153–54; paternalism in, 19, 41, 136

consent to treatment: advance directives on, 115–16; autonomy in, 43, 46, 115–16; by family or guardian, 5, 37–38, 122

consumers, use of term, 15

contracts: of family with hospital on lump sum payment, 125; household contract responsibility system, 34; psychiatric hospitals as prisons by contract, 40

control. See *guan*

Convention on the Rights of Persons with Disability (United Nations), 43

copresence, 81–82; shared delusions as, 79–80, 81

costs of treatment: in acute phase, 125; in community-based programs, 126; compared to income, 36, 138; contract agreements on, 40, 125; family responsibilities for, 4, 36, 65, 76, 125, 130, 138; government support in, 36, 125, 126; health insurance for (*see* health insurance); in long-term hospitalization, 76, 125; and profits, 36, 65–66; for psychopharmaceuticals, 36, 65, 125

counseling, 14

court cases on involuntary hospitalization: of Chen Dan, 29–31; hospital initiation of, 172n2; of Xu Wei, 2–4, 123–24, 126–29, 130–31, 160, 170–71n10

covert medications, 98–101, 102, 108

COVID-19 pandemic, 28, 157

Cultural Revolution, 33

culture: authority of parents in, 30; Confucian, 5; familial affection in, 48; gender roles in, 72–73; *guan* in, 54, 68, 131, 166n12; in Maoist era, 33; meaning systems in, 165n5; medical missionary view of, 8, 9, 10; natural task of caregiving in, 73, 138–39; paternalism in, 5, 6, 19, 31, 40, 41, 44, 47

danger: of endangering, 47, 111–12, 114; home confinement in, 91; involuntary hospitalization in, 43, 44, 47, 111–12, 114, 167n15

Das, Veena, 69, 152

Davis, Elizabeth, 112

deception by family caregivers, 97, 108; in covert medications, 98–101; in hospital admission, 1, 22, 67

decision-making on treatment: advance directives on, 115–16; autonomy in, 43, 46, 115–16; by family or guardian, 5, 37–38, 122; in medical protection hospitalization, 4, 37; supported, 161, 172n3

degeneration in mental illness, 62–63, 68, 71, 104

deinstitutionalization, 26, 38, 43, 45, 46, 158, 159

delusions, 37, 79–80, 81

dementia praecox, 62

dependency: caregiver view of, 151; as inherent human characteristic, 15–16, 135–36, 162; in quota scheme employment, 149; on state, 150, 159

depression, 29–30, 50; postpartum, 72

Derrida, Jacques, 98

diagnosis of mental illness: in being mentally illed, 41–43; in biomedical approach, 35; disorders included in, 14, 95; family reports as basis of, 22, 29, 30, 37, 58, 61; *guan* in management of, 18 (see also *guan*); guardianship in, 4 (*see also* guardianship); hospital-family circuit in, 31, 36–38; medical protection hospitalization in, 4, 30; Mental Health Law on, 44; personhood questioned in, 16; request for rediagnosis in, 43, 49; risk management in, 6 (*see also* risk management); in traditional Chinese medicine, 7, 37; in troublemakers and whistleblowers, 40

dibao (minimum living guarantee), 134, 137, 138, 140, 148

disability: abandonment of child with, 75, 156; certificate for transportation costs in, 133–34, 139; compassionate care in, 100; family caregivers in, 75–76, 140, 156; grave, involuntary hospitalization in, 170n5; intellectual, with psychosis, 14, 95; and "the old nurturing the disabled," 137–38, 140, 148, 151, 171n1; and one-child policy, 168n2; quota scheme employment in, 148–49, 171–72n6; risk assessment in, 121, 170n5; social security and health insurance in, 150–51; welfare benefits in, 139, 150

Disabled Persons' Federation, 135, 150

discharge from hospitalization, 123–29; autonomy rights in, 4, 124; family role in decisions on, 3, 4, 12, 30, 123, 124, 127–28, 160, 170n8; financial interests in, 113; guardian role in, 3, 127, 128; lawsuit on right to, 2–4, 123–24, 126–29, 160; of long-term patients, 123–29; Mental Health Law on, 111, 169n1 (chap. 5); patient requests for, 2–4, 40, 123–24, 126–29; return to work after, 2, 66, 72; violence risk in, 160; in voluntary admission, 128; of Xu Wei, 2–3, 124, 160–62

discipline, 8, 158, 162; by fathers, 82, 83, 105; in guan, 18, 54; in missionary psychiatry, 9

discrimination, 78; in disability, 139; in workplace, 74, 144, 145

disorganized behavior in self-disorder, 37

divorce, 76, 99

doctor-patient relationship, paternalism in, 41

domestic citizenship, 69, 70

Dong (Mrs.) and daughter Tingting. See Tingting and Mrs. Dong case example

Dumit, Joseph, 65

Duo (Sister), in "much joy" couple. See "much joy" couple

elderly, as caregivers. See aging caregivers

elderly, care for: family responsibilities in, 11; state promises of, in one-child policy, 140–41, 171n2

electroshock therapy, 33, 59, 117

emotions of family caregivers, 48, 143–46

employment: and dibao entitlements in unemployment, 148; discrimination in, 74, 144, 145; of family caregivers, 11, 134, 137, 139; quota scheme in, 148–49, 150, 171–72n6;

return to, after hospital discharge, 2, 66, 72; secret diagnosis of troublemakers in, 40, 41, 166n4; in state-owned enterprises, 11, 133, 137, 141; stress in, 2, 53, 74

England, 158

epilepsy with psychosis, 14, 95

Equity and Justice Initiative (EJI), 25, 26, 40, 166n5, 167n11

ethical issues: in guan, 17–19; in medical protection hospitalization, 37; in paternalism, 19; in risk calculations, 112, 113

eugenics, 9

exclusionary effects of SMIs, 71, 73–74, 75

familial affection (qinqing), 48

familial paternalism: aging caregivers in, 6, 84, 108, 134; coercion and deception in, 98, 108; culture of, 5, 31, 40, 41; global practices in, 6–7, 38, 157–58; guan in, 19, 27, 153; in market reform era, 38; Mental Health law on, 50; normalcy concept in, 84; recognition of caregiver labor in, 136, 153; scaling of, 32, 41, 49–50, 134, 150, 153; and state paternalism compared, 31, 32; state relegation of responsibilities to, 6–7, 50, 108, 134, 150, 160; women as caregivers in, 6, 20, 98, 108, 134

family: biopower of, 16, 17; configurations of, 6, 10; in Confucianism, 8, 10, 41; flexible positioning of, 89; found or chosen, 12, 163; and fragility of conjugality, 71–74; historical aspects of, 7–13, 32–36; in imperial China, 7–8, 11, 83–84, 88; in Maoist era, 10, 33; in market reform era, 11, 32, 34–35, 69, 71, 84, 88–90; as moral laboratory, 70

family caregivers, 1–13; abandonment by, 38, 76–77, 123, 128, 156; accommodation by, 12, 79–80, 83, 85; for adult children (see adult children, family responsibilities for); aging (see aging caregivers); art of disposition by, 67; authority of, 2, 22; avoidance by, 75; BeWell Family Resource Center for (see BeWell Family Resource Center); burden of care and suffering of, 48, 105–6, 144–46, 153; citizenship of, 136–37; compassion of (see compassion); consent to treatment by, 5, 37–38; copresence with patients, 81–82; deception in hospital admission by, 1, 22, 67; in discharge decisions, 3, 4, 12, 30, 123,

124, 127–28, 160, 170n8; as disciplinary agents, 8; education workshops for, 66–67, 117, 143–44; for elderly, 11, 140–41; emotions of, 48, 143–46; employment of, 11, 134, 137, 139; gendered patterns in roles of, 82–84 (*see also* gender); in *guan*, 2, 17–19 (see also *guan*); as guardians (*see* guardianship); home confinement by (*see* home confinement); involuntary hospitalization by, 5 (*see also* involuntary hospitalization); and kinship in serious mental illness, 69–85; legal responsibilities for homicide, 7–8; marginalization of (*see* marginalization of family caregivers); in medical protection hospitalization, 4; in medication compliance, 52, 53, 64–65, 82, 98–101; Mental Health Law on, 5, 18, 20, 31, 32, 39, 48–50, 117–20, 130; in natural task of caregiving, 35, 48, 65, 69, 73, 84; neglect by, 4; normalcy ideas of, 70, 83, 84–85; paternalistic responsibilities of (*see* familial paternalism); patient history reported by (*see* patient history, family reports of); payment of hospital costs by, 4, 36, 65, 76, 125, 130, 138; Qing laws on, 7–8; quests for order, 54–56; in relapse risk, 73, 112; research methodology on, 21–27; respite services for, 103, 104–5, 142; risk management by, 17, 20, 27, 48–49, 52–53, 64–68, 98; in sandwich class, 138; in 686 Program, 96–98; sociality of, 135, 145, 153; state expectations on self-sufficiency on, 139, 144; supplemental practices of (*see* supplemental practices, maternal); timely action by, 67; uncompensated labor of, 138, 143; in violence risk, 7–8, 98, 112, 134, 146–47, 152; vulnerability of, 150, 153; for vulnerable, 7, 15–16; welfare benefits for, 134, 137, 139; wrongful hospitalization by, 42, 48

family planning policies: change in, 156; on one child, 11, 69, 76, 140

family values, 13

Fan, Ruiping, 170n7

fear, 63, 68

feminism, on vulnerability and dependence as inherent characteristics, 15–16

filiality in Confucianism, 8, 10, 19, 154

foster care of disabled children, 156

Foucault, Michael, 166n10

Frazier, Mark, 171n3

freedom, personal, 118; and nonintervention decisions, 113–16; rights of patients to, 29; struggle of Wei for, 2–4, 160–62

fully human (*chengren*), 18

gender: and "cannot bear," 105–6; of caregivers, 11, 12, 90 (*see also* men, as caregivers; women, as caregivers); and chaotic experiences, 55–56; and compassion, 12, 83–84, 105–6; and Confucian values on male domination, 11; and exclusionary effects of SMIs, 73–74; and normalcy concept of parents, 82–84; and paternalism, 20, 166n13; of patients (*see* men, as patients; women, as patients); and power in imperial China, 11

genetics, 9, 59, 73, 168n5 (chap. 2)

ghosts, visions of, 52, 54, 58, 66

Giddens, Anthony, 112

Ginsburg, Faye, 70

Goffman, Erving, 12, 53

gong quanli (public power), 41

Good, Mary-Jo DelVecchio, 65

Greenhouse, Carol, 169–70n2

guakao, in quota scheme employment, 149, 150

guan, 17–19, 61, 130–31, 155; for adult child, 2, 18, 54, 61, 74, 76, 127; biopolitical vision of, 107; burden for caregiver in, 107, 146–47; cultural meaning of, 54, 68, 131, 166n12; historical requirement for, 8; importance and prevalence of, 166n12; in indefinite long-term hospitalization, 76, 77–78, 84, 131; in involuntary hospitalization, 17, 19, 61–62, 67, 119, 127, 130–31; in medication compliance, 65; Mental Health Law on, 18, 46, 118, 130–31; as nourishing or suffocating, 163; and order, 18, 56, 61, 68, 108; and paternalism, 19, 27, 41, 98, 108, 134, 150, 153; polysemous concept of, 17–18, 153; in risk management, 27, 97, 98, 120, 130; scaling idea of, 134; in 686 program, 96, 97, 98; state responsibilities of, 117, 119, 147, 149, 154; for vulnerable children, 18, 54; for Xu Wei, 3, 19, 127, 130–31, 160

guanli (supervision and management), 18, 46, 56

guansuo (chained or locked up), 101

guardianship, 12, 30, 126–28; abandonment in, 128; autonomy in, 49; consent to treatment in, 5, 37; hospitalization decisions in, 3, 4, 5, 49, 124, 126–28; Mental Health Law on, 5, 31, 49; paternalism in, 157; of Xu Wei, 2, 3, 17, 124, 126–27, 160

guojia fuquan, 5. *See also* state paternalism

hallucinations: in abortion and lack of marital recognition, 56, 71; ghostly visions in, 52, 54, 58, 66; in self-disorder, 37
Haraway, Donna, 21
He Jiyue, 87
health: concept of, 65; right to, 30, 31, 45–46, 47
health insurance, 33, 34; for hospitalization, 3, 4, 76, 125, 138; knowledge of caregivers on, 145; maximum annual benefits paid, 142; for medications, 36; in psychiatric disabilities, 150–51; public, 3, 4, 34, 36, 76, 125, 138, 148; in quota scheme employment, 149; for sanatorium stay of family caregivers, 142
heart, knotted, in schizophrenia and thought struggles, 80
Hedgecoe, Adam, 168n5 (chap. 2)
Hoffman, Browning, 167n14
home confinement, 87–88, 91–95, 101–7; burden of, 105–7, 108; community mental health services in, 88, 89; definition of, 103; free inpatient stay for caregiver respite in, 103, 104–5; history of, 8, 9, 88; images of, 92f, 93f; in Japan, 101, 106, 158; *New York Times* article on, 87–88, 91, 168–69n1; resistance to unlocking effort in, 94, 94f; risk management in, 91, 94–95, 103–4, 106–7; Unlock Action in, 88, 92, 95, 96
homeless people, 158, 159
home visits: by CMHPs, 96–103, 107, 120; and nonintervention in autonomy concerns, 113–16; in 686 Program, 96–97
homicide, family responsibility for, 7–8
hope for recovery, 63, 68, 70, 72, 123; in biomedicine, 56; of caregivers, 54, 77, 83; of doctors, 72; and fear of degeneration, 63, 68; and freedom, 123–24
Hopper, Kim, 166n3
hospital-family circuit of mental health care, 12, 31, 36–38, 53, 67–68, 116–17
hospitalization: as abandonment, 38, 76–77, 123, 128; advertisement on benefits of,

56–57, 57f, 62; advice to family on, 4, 37; authority of family in decisions on, 2; autonomy in, 4, 31, 114–16, 124; for bipolar disorder, 1–2, 172n2; cost of, 3, 4, 34, 36, 65, 76, 125, 138; deception of family about, 1–2, 22, 67; discharge from (*see* discharge from hospitalization); family visits during, 61–62; financial interests in, 36, 40, 66, 113, 124–26; free, 103–5; guardian decisions on, 3, 4, 5, 49, 124, 126–28; of homeless people, 159; hope for freedom from, 123–24; indefinite and long-term (*see* indefinite and long-term hospitalization); involuntary (*see* involuntary hospitalization); medical protection, 4, 30, 31, 37, 44; number of beds available for, 10, 33, 36, 45, 104, 126; order in, 60–61; and rehospitalization decisions, 66, 104, 126; reluctance of family about, 103, 104–5; routine use and legal expectation of, 14; in timely manner, 67; turnover rate of patients in, 125; voluntary (*see* voluntary hospitalization); wrongful (*see* wrongful hospitalization)
household contract responsibility system, 34
household registration status (*hukou*), 76, 140
Huan (Uncle), in "much joy" couple. *See* "much joy" couple
Huang Xuetao, 30, 39–40, 41, 167n6; on "being mentally illed" cases, 42–43; on patient autonomy and advance directives, 115–16; on right to health, 46; and Xu Wei, 3, 5, 123–24, 128–29, 170–71n10
hukou (household registration status), 76, 140
human rights activists, 26; on autonomy and right to health, 46; on being mentally illed, 31, 42–43; Huang Xuetao as, 3, 5, 30, 39–40, 41; on involuntary hospitalization, 5, 30, 31, 39–44, 123–24, 128–29; on long-term hospitalization, 123–24; on paternalism, 5, 19, 50

identity, collective, of caregivers, 146
imperial China, 7–8, 11, 83–84; filiality in, 10; home confinement in, 8, 88; madness concept in, 7–8
improvisations, 12, 13
income: compared to treatment costs, 36, 138; in minimum living guarantee (*dibao*), 134, 137, 138, 140, 148; in quota scheme employment, 149, 150; from retirement pensions, 137, 160

Peng Baoquan, 41, 42

"people, the," reconfigured as the population, 6, 89, 156

People's Republic, 10, 11, 12, 32

peri-urban hospitals, 125–26

perphenazine, covert administration of, 99, 100

Perry, Elizabeth, 151

personality: accommodation of, 79–80, 83; familiar, lost in mental illness, 81

personhood in SMI diagnosis, 16

Phillips, Michael, 167n11

"pick-up" services of hospitals, 44, 67, 114, 116, 117

Pinto, Sarah, 69, 77

police, role of: in arrest and hospitalization, 40; in employee being mentally illed, 41, 48; in Kerr Refuge admissions, 9; and nonintervention in liability concerns, 113, 114, 116; in release from hospital, 39; and requests for rediagnosis, 49; in risk management, 111, 114, 117–18, 121, 122; in transportation to hospital, 116, 120, 122

polygamy, 10

polysemy of *guan*, 17–18, 153

Pool, Deborah, 152

poorhouses, 158

population crisis, 156

population management, 6, 89, 107; biopolitical task of, 98, 105; coercive edge of, 104, 105; in eugenics, 9; and reconfiguration of "the people," 6, 89, 156; 686 Program in, 96

postpartum depression, 72

power, 22; in biopower and care, 15–17; public and oppressive, 41

prisons by contract (*qiyue jianyu*), 40

privatization, 15, 20, 36, 88, 90

profits, 36, 65, 66

prognosis in mental illness, 62–63, 104; and degeneration, 62–63, 68, 71, 104; and market calculations, 71–72; and relapse risk (*see* relapse risk)

Program for Managing and Treating Serious Mental Illnesses, 95. *See also* 686 Program

psychiatric hospitals: and deinstitutionalization, 43; financial interests of, 36, 66, 124–26; in market reform era, 34–38; number of beds in, 10, 33, 36, 45, 104, 126; "pick-up" services of, 44, 67, 114, 116, 117; as prisons

by contract, 40; research methodology on, 21–22; rural and peri-urban, 125–26; as total institutions, 12; turnover rate of patients in, 125. *See also* hospitalization

psychiatrists: on advance directives, 115–16; advising on hospitalization decisions, 4, 37; on autonomy and right to health, 46; being mentally illed by, 42; in drafting Mental Health Law, 5, 25, 34, 38–39, 44–45, 47, 48, 118; on emotions of caregivers, 143; forensic, 38, 40, 45, 160; on insight and self-disorder, 36–37; on involuntary hospitalization, 5, 31; on long-term hospitalization, 124–25; in market reform era, 35–36; on medical protection hospitalization, 31; number in China, 10, 33, 36; on paternalism, 5, 19; on risk criteria, 119, 120–21; in secret diagnosis of troublemakers, 40, 166n4; on suicide in nonintervention, 114–15, 116, 119, 120

psychiatry: abuse of (*see* abuse, psychiatric); biomedical (*see* biomedical psychiatry); claims on benefits of, 57, 59, 62, 104; globalization and selective adaptation of, 165n7; historical development of, 7–10, 33–36; missionary, 8–9, 31–32, 88; professionalization of, 35; as quick fix, 62, 64, 68; research methodology on, 21–27

psychopharmaceutical treatment, 13–14, 59–60; coercion in, 14, 98–101; compliance with (*see* compliance with medications); cost of, 36, 65, 125; covert, 98–101; historical aspects of, 33, 35; in home confinement, 102, 104; in neurochemical imbalances, 13, 35, 59; phases of, 62; in risk management, 64–66, 68, 72, 99; in schizophrenia, 62, 79, 80, 99–100, 102; side effects of, 35, 52, 59–60, 64, 73, 100; in 686 Program, 96, 97, 104, 169n5; symptom management in, 62, 79

psychosis, 14, 40, 95

psychosociality, 145

psychotherapy, 35

public harm, risk of, 97, 104, 116, 122

public health system, 91

public housing: BeWell services for community in, 24, 133; and biopolitical paternalism in US, 159; marginal households in, 137; qualifications for, 144, 147

public power (*gong quanli*), 41

service users, use of term, 15
sex: with insane as forbidden, 9; and male
    patients seen as sexually overactive, 74;
    parent listening to imagined details about,
    81–82; and unfulfilled desires as cause of
    madness, 7
Shao, Yang, 170n6
Simonis, Fabien, 8
Sina Weibo, 41, 167n6
sister, use of term, 168n6 (chap. 3)
Sister Duo in "much joy" couple. *See* "much
    joy" couple
situated knowledges, 21
686 Program, 88, 89, 90, 91, 95–98; commu-
    nity mental health practitioners (CMHPS)
    in, 96–97, 120; home confinement in, 101,
    103; levels of risk in, 97, 104, 120, 121; medi-
    cations in, 96, 97, 104, 169n5; public risk as
    concern in, 97, 104, 116; state funding of,
    96; violence risk as concern in, 95–98, 106,
    107–8, 116
sleep problems, 1, 53, 54, 58, 63
social construction of madness/mental illness,
    13–15
socialist institutions and practices, 19, 20; in-
    voluntary interventions in, 20; paternalism
    in, 47, 50, 90, 118, 136, 151, 156, 159; speaking
    bitterness in, 145–46
sociality of family caregivers, 134, 145, 153
socialization, 18
social membership, indefinite hospitalization
    affecting, 17, 77, 84
social reproduction, 32, 74, 84
social security, 141, 148, 149, 150–51
social work agencies, 13
speaking bitterness (*suku*), 145–46
Spears, Britney, 158
stability maintenance (*weiwen*), 95, 96, 147
stabilization phase of treatment, 62
State Council, 39, 44, 49
state-owned enterprises, 136; loss of jobs in, 11,
    133, 137, 141; in market reform era, 34, 137;
    retirement pensions from, 11, 141, 171n3;
    structural adjustment of, 141
state paternalism, 5, 19, 20, 27–28, 30, 41; adult
    patient care in, 147–48; dependence on,
    159; desire of caregivers and patients for,
    162; and family paternalism compared, 31,
    32; fear of potential overreach in, 20–21,

50; involuntary hospitalization in, 32; in
    Maoist era, 32, 33–34, 47, 136; in market
    reform era, 136; Mental Health Law on, 5,
    20, 46–47, 50, 118–19; and right to health,
    44–47; scaling of, 32, 41, 49–50, 150, 153;
    socialist, 47, 50, 118, 136, 151, 156, 159; in
    work units, 148, 149
state roles and responsibilities: for adult
    patients, 147–48; caregiver dependency
    in, 150; in COVID-19 pandemic, 157; and
    expectations of self-sufficiency, 139, 144; of
    guan, 117, 119, 147, 149, 154; hypocrisy in,
    141, 152, 157; in Maoist regime, 10, 11; and
    marginalization of family caregivers, 135,
    136, 137, 138, 141; in market reform era, 11,
    89, 136; Mental Health Law on, 5, 20, 47; in
    neoliberalism, 50, 138, 142; as parent, 6, 32,
    33, 89, 96, 107, 108, 147, 149; in paternalism
    (*see* state paternalism); in security, 6, 156; in
    686 Program, 89, 96; in socialist traditions,
    19, 50; in stability maintenance, 95, 147; in
    violence risk, 146–47
Steinmüller, Hans, 142, 171n4
stigma of mental illness, 74; by association, 75;
    in biomedical psychiatry, 14; and burden
    of care in family, 48; caregiver advocacy af-
    fecting, 153; and family refusal of discharge,
    123; in medication side effects, 64; in
    schizophrenia of parent, 21
stress: and genetic factors in mental illness, 59,
    168n5 (chap. 2); as precipitating factor, 64;
    in workplace, 2, 53
subaltern status, 98, 108
suffering, 15; of family caregivers, 144–46, 150,
    153; of household in home confinement,
    106; speaking bitterness in, 145–46; as
    unbearable, compassion in, 104–7
suicidal behavior, 3; autonomy and nonin-
    tervention in, 113–16, 117, 119; and being
    suicided, 41; of rural women in Northern
    China, 168n3 (chap. 2)
suku (speaking bitterness), 145–46
Sun Dongdong, 40, 46, 47
supplemental practices, maternal, 27, 162–63;
    in biopolitical paternalism, 98, 101, 106,
    107–9; covert medication as, 98–101; in
    vulnerability of patient and caregiver, 20
supported decision-making, 161, 172n3
survivors, use of term, 15

women, as patients (*continued*)
with, 81–82; family reports on, 58, 66, 73; ghostly visions of, 52, 54, 58, 66; involuntary hospitalization of, 39–40, 158; long-term hospitalization of, 77; medication side effects and noncompliance in, 52, 60, 73; in "much joy" couple (*see* "much joy" couple); refusal to visit natal home, 58–59, 73; relapse risk in, 52, 73; risk management in, 52–53, 68; in schizophrenia, 58–59, 78–80, 99–100, 138, 139; Tingting as (*see* Tingting and Mrs. Dong case example)

workplace. *See* employment

work therapy in Maoist era, 33

work units, 10, 33; end of, 88; role in involuntary hospitalization, 48, 114; state paternalism in, 148, 149; wages and benefits in, 141

World Health Organization, 39, 44, 45

wrongful hospitalization, 24, 43–44; in being mentally illed, 30, 42, 43, 45; family role in, 42, 48; legal issues in, 42, 43, 45, 112, 113–16, 117; and nonintervention protecting patient autonomy, 113–16; number of cases involving, 40, 118, 166n5; release from, 123; scaling of issues in, 43–44, 45; as systemic psychiatric abuse, 43–44

Wu, Fei, 168n3 (chap. 2)

Xi Jinping, 118, 156

xiaoxin kanguan (carefully watched over), 3

Xie, Bin, 170n6

Xu Wei, 2–4, 123–24, 126–29, 160–62, 170–71n10; discharge from hospital, 2–3, 124, 160–62; girlfriend of, 160, 161, 172n1; *guan* for, 3, 19, 127, 130–31, 160; guardian of, 2, 3, 17, 124, 126–27, 160; and Huang Xuetao, 3, 5, 123–24, 128–29, 170–71n10; indefinite hospitalization of, 17, 19; involuntary hospitalization of, 2–4, 123–24, 126–28, 129, 130–31

Yan Jun, 90–91

Yan, Yunxiang, 11

Yu Xin, 126, 167n13

zero COVID policy, 157

Zhang Dejiang, 34–35

Zhang, Li, 145

Zhang, Yonghong, 147

zhi (treating or curing disease), 168n4 (chap. 2)

Zhu, Jianfeng, 166n12

zizhili (insight), 36–37, 44

Zou Yijun, 39–40

www.ingramcontent.com/pod-product-compliance
Lightning Source LLC
Chambersburg PA
CBHW030822270326
41928CB00007B/858